The Complete
Air Fryer Cookbook

Delicious and Healthy Recipes to Cook for
the Whole Family using the Air Fryer

Martine Haley

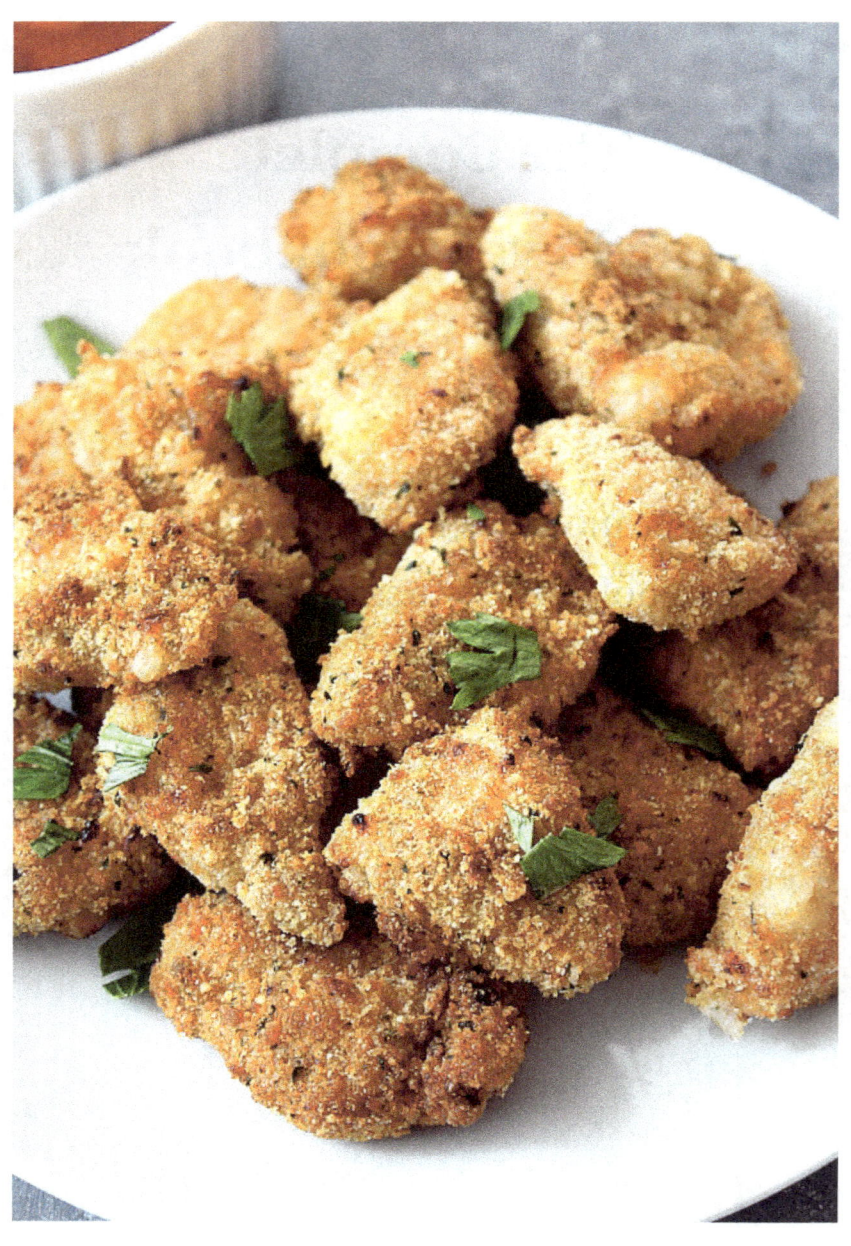

Table of Contents

—

INTRODUCTION

An air fryer is a kitchen appliance designed to deliver a tasty, crispy, golden-brown morsel of food without the use of oil or other cooking fats. It uses hot air instead of oil or other cooking fats to cook food quickly and evenly.

The air fryer can be used for making fried chips in addition to other foods.

There are several varieties of air fryers. One of the main categories is made up of countertop air fryers designed for individual use in the kitchen. These models sit on the worktop or counter top and feature a basket that sits on a wire rack. This forms the base that holds hot air that cooks food as it passes through it.

air fryer's air fryers are designed to help you make healthy and filling meals. Our electric fryers are perfect for people who want fresh, homemade fries without all of the fat. Our air fryer features a light-weight aluminum design that lets you move the appliance from room to room without worry. Each air fryer is also equipped with a thermostat, making it easy to adjust the temperature as needed.

An air fryer is an appliance that cooks food using high-speed air circulation. It is a perfect alternative to deep frying, baking or roasting, and works great for cooking fast and healthy meals.

How Does an Air Fryer Work?

The fan draws warm air from the bottom of the chamber, which rises and cools as it circulates. The food is then placed in the middle of the basket, and the fan circulates air around it, cooking it all at once. Food cooks faster than if you fried it in oil or baked it in an oven. The food doesn't become soggy like fried food does, either. Because the air circulates around the food rather than through it, you can use much less oil in your Air Fryer. Best of all, since no oil is being used for cooking, there's much less of an environmental impact!

What Types of Air Fryers are Available?

Air fryers come in a variety of sizes as well as different colors and designs. You may find one that has a View Master-like chrome trim or one with a retro design pattern that blends easily into your décor. Some Air fryers are as small as a rice cooker while others can be used to make large batches of French fries with recipes you create on your tablet! Some Air Fryer models have "smart" features that allow you to cook multiple foods at the same time; others have timers so you can automatically set them for particular times during the day. All versions sterilize their own cooking plates by running them through a clean cycle between batches!

When you are looking for a new air fryer, you should take a look at air fryer Cookware. We have all of the features you are looking for in an air fryer, including built in racks that will allow you to cook a full size meal for your family. We also have a variety of accessories that will give you an even better cooking experience.

We are proud to introduce air fryer Cookware, the premier brand in air fryers. You can rest assured that we only use the best materials to ensure our products will work for years to come. Our air fryers feature built-in racks, so you can cook a full-size meal at once. They also include an adjustable thermostat that ranges from 120 to 500 degrees Fahrenheit.

Whether you are looking to impress your family with gourmet French fries or just want to make your favorite chicken drumsticks and vegetables, air fryer Cookware has everything you need. Every item has been carefully tested to ensure safe and responsible use. All of our products carry a One Year Limited Manufacturer Warranty, so you can be confident that they will serve your needs well.

BBQ Pork Chops

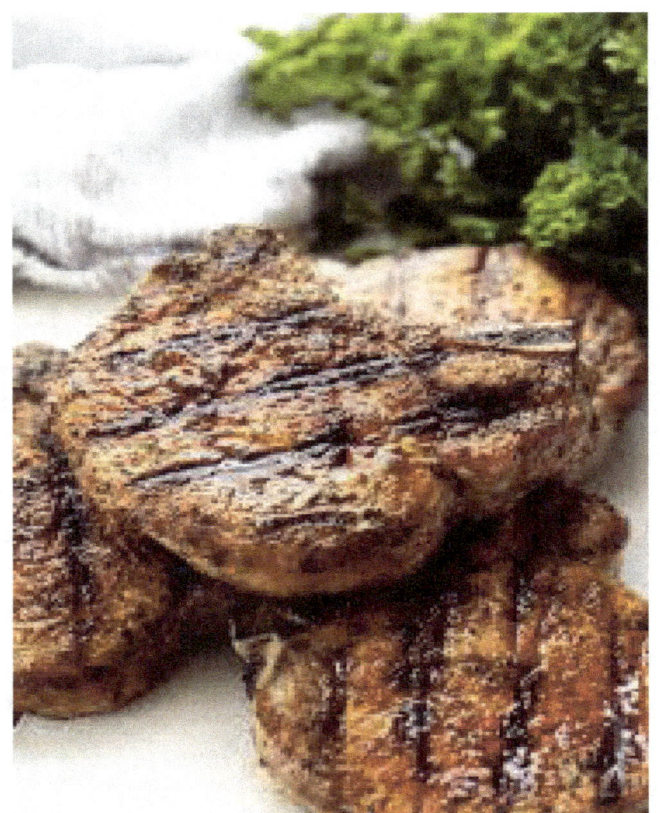

Basic Recipe
Preparation Time: 10 minutes
Cooking Time: 7 minutes
Servings: 4
Ingredients:
- 4 pork chops
- For rub:
- ½ tsp allspice
- ½ tsp dry mustard
- 1 tsp ground cumin
- 1 tsp garlic powder

- ½ tsp chili powder
- ½ tsp paprika
- 1 tbsp brown sugar
- 1 tsp salt

Directions:

1. In a small bowl, mix together all rub ingredients and rub all over pork chops.
2. Arrange pork chops on air fryer tray and air fry at 400 F for 5.
3. Turn pork chops to other side and air fry for 2 minutes more.
4. Serve and enjoy.

Nutrition: Calories 273 Fat 20.2 g Carbs 3.4 g Protein 18.4 g

Simple Beef Patties

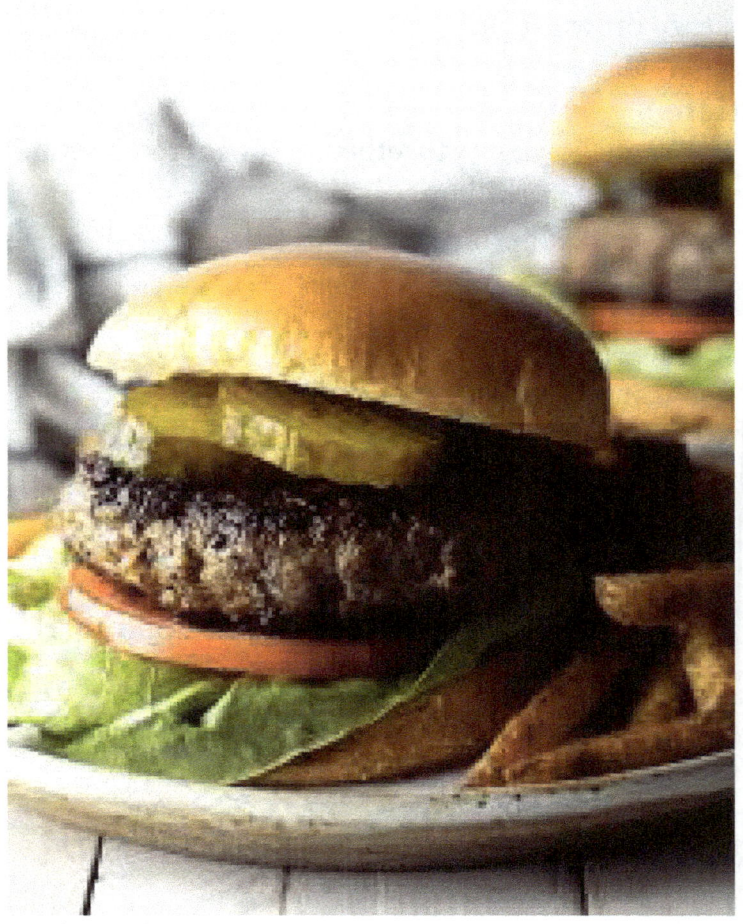

Basic Recipe
Preparation Time: 10 minutes
Cooking Time: 13 minutes
Servings: 4
Ingredients:
- 1 lb. ground beef
- ½ tsp garlic powder
- ¼ tsp onion powder

- Pepper
- Salt

Directions:

1. Preheat the instant vortex air fryer oven to 400 F.
2. Add ground meat, garlic powder, onion powder, pepper, and salt into the mixing bowl and mix until well combined.
3. Make even shape patties from meat mixture and arrange on air fryer pan.
4. Place pan in instant vortex air fryer oven.
5. Cook patties for 10 minutes Turn patties after 5 minutes
6. Serve and enjoy.

Nutrition: Calories 212 Fat 7.1 g Carbs 0.4 g Protein 34.5 g

Simple Beef Sirloin Roast

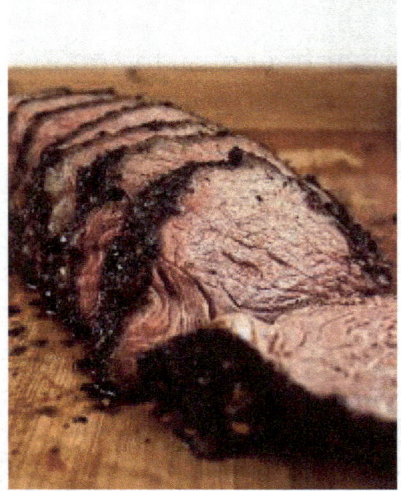

Basic Recipe
Preparation Time: 10 minutes
Cooking Time: 50 minutes
Servings: 8

Ingredients:

- 2½ pounds sirloin roast
- Salt and ground black pepper, as required

Directions:

1. Rub the roast with salt and black pepper generously.
2. Insert the rotisserie rod through the roast.
3. Insert the rotisserie forks, one on each side of the rod to secure the rod to the chicken.
4. Arrange the drip pan in the bottom of Instant Vortex Plus Air Fryer Oven cooking chamber.
5. Select "Roast" and then adjust the temperature to 350 degrees F.
6. Set the timer for 50 minutes and press the "Start".

7. When the display shows "Add Food" press the red lever down and load the left side of the rod into the Vortex.
8. Now, slide the rod's left side into the groove along the metal bar so it doesn't move. Then, close the door and touch "Rotate". Press the red lever to release the rod when cooking time is complete.
9. Remove from the Vortex and place the roast onto a platter for about 10 minutes before slicing. With a sharp knife, cut the roast into desired sized slices and serve.

Nutrition: Calories 201 Fat 8.8 g Carbs 0 g Protein 28.9 g

Seasoned Beef Roast

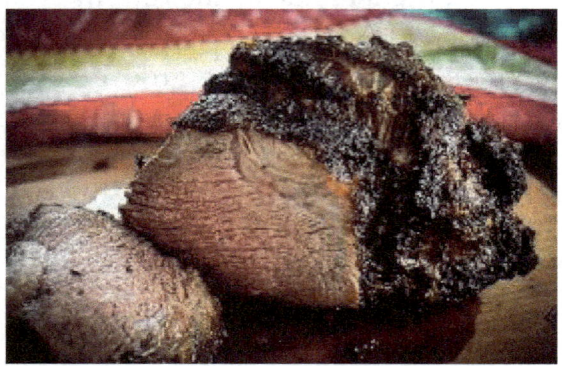

Basic Recipe
Preparation Time: 10 minutes
Cooking Time: 45 minutes
Servings: 10

Ingredients:

- 3 pounds beef top roast
- 1 tablespoon olive oil
- 2 tablespoons Montreal steak seasoning

Directions:

1. Coat the roast with oil and then rub with the seasoning generously.
2. With kitchen twines, tie the roast to keep it compact. Arrange the roast onto the cooking tray.
3. Arrange the drip pan in the bottom of Instant Vortex plus Air Fryer Oven cooking chamber.
4. Select "Air Fry" and then adjust the temperature to 360 degrees F. Set the timer for 45 minutes and press the "Start".
5. When the display shows "Add Food" insert the cooking tray in the center position.
6. When the display shows "Turn Food" do nothing.

7. When cooking time is complete, remove the tray from Vortex and place the roast onto a platter for about 10 minutes before slicing. With a sharp knife, cut the roast into desired sized slices and serve.

Nutrition: Calories 269 Fat 9.9 g Carbs 0 g Fiber 0 g

Bacon Wrapped Filet Mignon

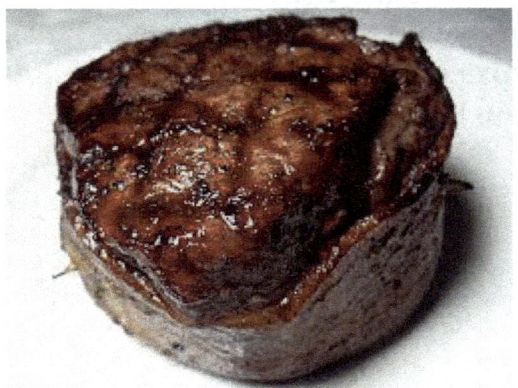

Basic Recipe
Preparation Time: 10 minutes
Cooking Time: 15 minutes
Servings: 2

Ingredients:

- 2 bacon slices
- 2 (4-ounce) filet mignon
- Salt and ground black pepper, as required
- Olive oil cooking spray

Directions:

1. Wrap 1 bacon slice around each filet mignon and secure with toothpicks.
2. Season the filets with the salt and black pepper lightly.
3. Arrange the filet mignon onto a coking rack and spray with cooking spray.
4. Arrange the drip pan in the bottom of Instant Vortex plus Air Fryer Oven cooking chamber.
5. Select "Air Fry" and then adjust the temperature to 375 degrees F.
6. Set the timer for 15 minutes and press the "Start".

7. When the display shows "Add Food" insert the cooking rack in the center position.
8. When the display shows "Turn Food" turn the filets.
9. When cooking time is complete, remove the rack from Vortex and serve hot.

Nutrition: Calories 360 Fat 19.6 g Carbs 0.4 g Protein 42.6 g

Beef Burgers

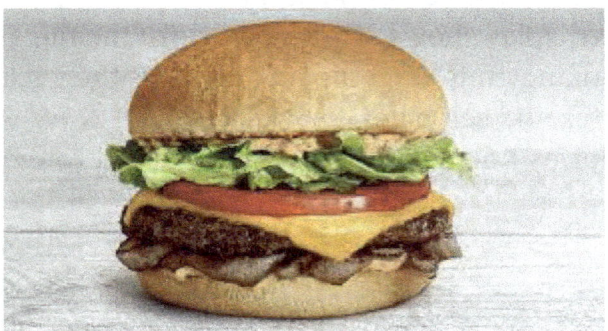

Basic Recipe
Preparation Time: 15 minutes
Cooking Time: 18 minutes
Servings: 4

Ingredients:

- For Burgers:
- 1-pound ground beef
- ½ cup panko breadcrumbs
- ¼ cup onion, chopped finely
- 3 tablespoons Dijon mustard
- 3 teaspoons low-sodium soy sauce
- 2 teaspoons fresh rosemary, chopped finely
- Salt, to taste
- For Topping:
- 2 tablespoons Dijon mustard
- 1 tablespoon brown sugar
- 1 teaspoon soy sauce
- 4 Gruyere cheese slices

Directions:

1. In a large bowl, add all the ingredients and mix until well combined.
2. Make 4 equal-sized patties from the mixture.

3. Arrange the patties onto a cooking tray.
4. Arrange the drip pan in the bottom of Instant Vortex Plus Air Fryer Oven cooking chamber.
5. Select "Air Fry" and then adjust the temperature to 370 degrees F.
6. Set the timer for 15 minutes and press the "Start".
7. When the display shows "Add Food" insert the cooking rack in the center position.
8. When the display shows "Turn Food" turn the burgers.
9. Meanwhile, for sauce: in a small bowl, add the mustard, brown sugar and soy sauce and mix well.
10. When cooking time is complete, remove the tray from Vortex and coat the burgers with the sauce.
11. Top each burger with 1 cheese slice.
12. Return the tray to the cooking chamber and select "Broil".
13. Set the timer for 3 minutes and press the "Start".
14. When cooking time is complete, remove the tray from Vortex and serve hot.

Nutrition: Calories 402 Fat 18 g Carbs 6.3 g Protein 44.4 g

Season and Salt-Cured Beef

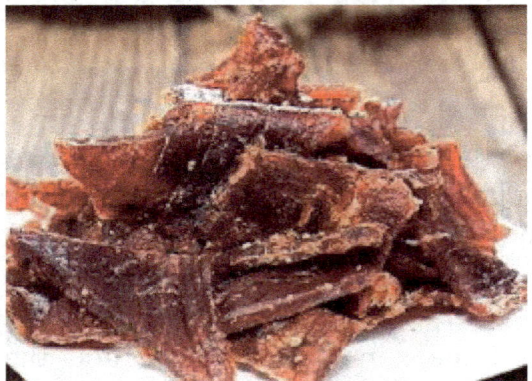

Intermediate Recipe
Preparation Time: 15 minutes
Cooking Time: 3 hours
Servings: 4

Ingredients:

- 1½ pounds beef round, trimmed
- ½ cup Worcestershire sauce
- ½ cup low-sodium soy sauce
- 2 teaspoons honey
- 1 teaspoon liquid smoke
- 2 teaspoons onion powder
- ½ teaspoon red pepper flakes
- Ground black pepper, as required

Directions:

1. In a zip-top bag, place the beef and freeze for 1-2 hours to firm up.
2. Place the meat onto a cutting board and cut against the grain into 1/8-¼-inch strips.
3. In a large bowl, add the remaining ingredients and mix until well combined.

4. Add the steak slices and coat with the mixture generously.
5. Refrigerate to marinate for about 4-6 hours.
6. Remove the beef slices from bowl and with paper towels, pat dry them.
7. Divide the steak strips onto the cooking trays and arrange in an even layer.
8. Select "Dehydrate" and then adjust the temperature to 160 degrees F.
9. Set the timer for 3 hours and press the "Start".
10. When the display shows "Add Food" insert 1 tray in the top position and another in the center position.
11. After 1½ hours, switch the position of cooking trays.
12. Meanwhile, in a small pan, add the remaining ingredients over medium heat and cook for about 10 minutes, stirring occasionally.
13. When cooking time is complete, remove the trays from Vortex.

Nutrition: Calories 372 Fat 10.7 g Carbs 12 g Protein 53.8 g

Sweet & Spicy Meatballs

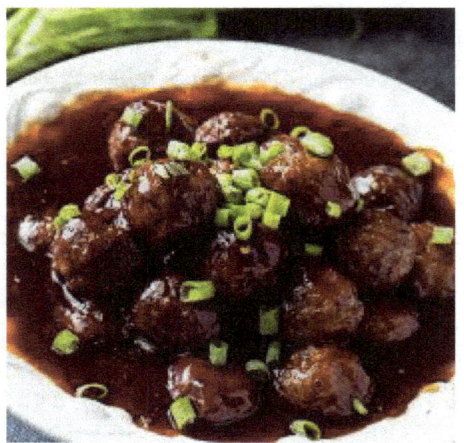

Basic Recipe
Preparation Time: 20 minutes
Cooking Time: 30 minutes
Servings: 8

Ingredients:

- For Meatballs:
- 2 pounds lean ground beef
- 2/3 cup quick-cooking oats
- ½ cup Ritz crackers, crushed
- 1 (5-ounce) can evaporated milk
- 2 large eggs, beaten lightly
- 1 teaspoon honey
- 1 tablespoon dried onion, minced
- 1 teaspoon garlic powder
- 1 teaspoon ground cumin
- Salt and ground black pepper, as required
- For Sauce:
- 1/3 cup orange marmalade
- 1/3 cup honey

- 1/3 cup brown sugar
- 2 tablespoons cornstarch
- 2 tablespoons soy sauce
- 1-2 tablespoons hot sauce
- 1 tablespoon Worcestershire sauce

Directions:

1. For meatballs: in a large bowl, add all the ingredients and mix until well combined.
2. Make 1½-inch balls from the mixture.
3. Arrange half of the meatballs onto a cooking tray in a single layer.
4. Arrange the drip pan in the bottom of Instant Vortex Plus Air Fryer Oven cooking chamber.
5. Select "Air Fry" and then adjust the temperature to 380 degrees F.
6. Set the timer for 15 minutes and press the "Start".
7. When the display shows "Add Food" insert the cooking tray in the center position.
8. When the display shows "Turn Food" turn the meatballs.
9. When cooking time is complete, remove the tray from Vortex.
10. Repeat with the remaining meatballs.
11. Meanwhile, for sauce: in a small pan, add all the ingredients over medium heat and cook until thickened, stirring continuously.
12. Serve the meatballs with the topping of sauce.

Nutrition: Calories 411 Fat 11.1 g Carbs 38.8 g Protein 38.9 g

Spiced Pork Shoulder

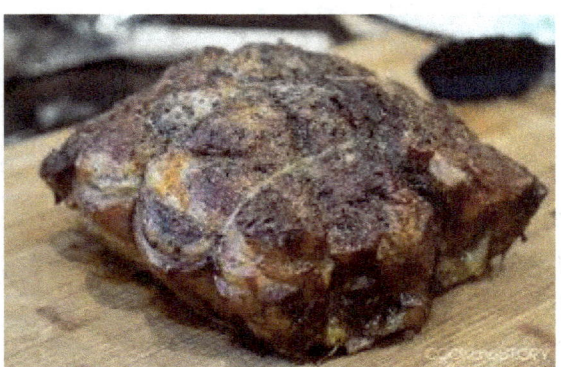

Basic Recipe
Preparation Time: 15 minutes
Cooking Time: 55 minutes
Servings: 6

Ingredients:

- 1 teaspoon ground cumin
- 1 teaspoon cayenne pepper
- 1 teaspoon garlic powder
- Salt and ground black pepper, as required
- 2 pounds skin-on pork shoulder

Directions:

1. In a small bowl, mix together the spices, salt and black pepper.
2. Arrange the pork shoulder onto a cutting board, skin-side down.
3. Season the inner side of pork shoulder with salt and black pepper.
4. With kitchen twines, tie the pork shoulder into a long round cylinder shape.
5. Season the outer side of pork shoulder with spice mixture.
6. Insert the rotisserie rod through the pork shoulder.

7. Insert the rotisserie forks, one on each side of the rod to secure the pork shoulder.
8. Arrange the drip pan in the bottom of Instant Vortex Plus Air Fryer Oven cooking chamber.
9. Select "Roast" and then adjust the temperature to 350 degrees F.
10. Set the timer for 55 minutes and press the 'Start".
11. When the display shows "Add Food" press the red lever down and load the left side of the rod into the Vortex.
12. Now, slide the rod's left side into the groove along the metal bar so it doesn't move.
13. Then, close the door and touch "Rotate".
14. Press the red lever to release the rod when cooking time is complete.
15. Remove the pork from Vortex and place onto a platter for about 10 minutes before slicing.
16. With a sharp knife, cut the pork shoulder into desired sized slices and serve.

Nutrition: Calories 445 Fat 32.5 g Carbs 0.7 g Protein 35.4 g

Seasoned Pork Tenderloin

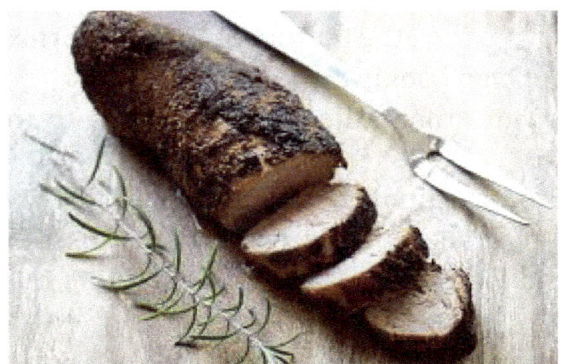

Basic Recipe
Preparation Time: 10 minutes
Cooking Time: 45 minutes
Servings: 5

Ingredients:

- 1½ pounds pork tenderloin
- 2-3 tablespoons BBQ pork seasoning

Directions:

1. Rub the pork with seasoning generously.Insert the rotisserie rod through the pork tenderloin.
2. Insert the rotisserie forks, one on each side of the rod to secure the pork tenderloin.
3. Arrange the drip pan in the bottom of Instant Vortex plus Air Fryer Oven cooking chamber.
4. Select "Roast" and then adjust the temperature to 360 degrees F.
5. Set the timer for 45 minutes and press the "Start".
6. When the display shows "Add Food" press the red lever down and load the left side of the rod into the Vortex.
7. Now, slide the rod's left side into the groove along the metal bar so it doesn't move.

8. Then, close the door and touch "Rotate".
9. Press the red lever to release the rod when cooking time is complete.
10. Remove the pork from Vortex and place onto a platter for about 10 minutes before slicing.
11. With a sharp knife, cut the roast into desired sized slices and serve.

Nutrition: Calories 195 Fat 4.8 g Carbs 0 g Protein 35.6 g

Garlicky Pork Tenderloin

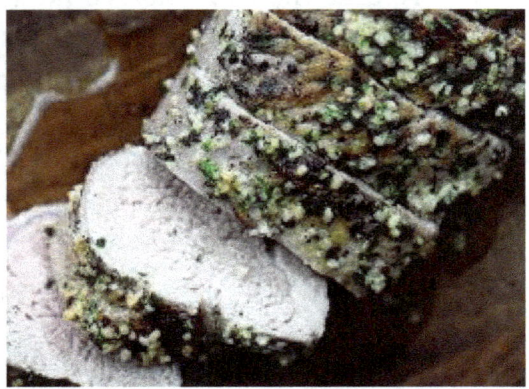

Basic Recipe
Preparation Time: 15 minutes
Cooking Time: 20 minutes
Servings: 5

Ingredients:

- 1½ pounds pork tenderloin
- Nonstick cooking spray
- 2 small heads roasted garlic
- Salt and ground black pepper, as required

Directions:

1. Lightly, spray all the sides of pork with cooking spray and then, season with salt and black pepper.
2. Now, rub the pork with roasted garlic. Arrange the roast onto the lightly greased cooking tray.
3. Arrange the drip pan in the bottom of Instant Vortex plus Air Fryer Oven cooking chamber.
4. Select "Air Fry" and then adjust the temperature to 400 degrees F. Set the timer for 20 minutes and press the "Start".
5. When the display shows "Add Food" insert the cooking tray in the center position.

―

6. When the display shows "Turn Food" turn the pork.
7. When cooking time is complete, remove the tray from Vortex and place the roast onto a platter for about 10 minutes before slicing. With a sharp knife, cut the roast into desired sized slices and serve.

Nutrition: Calories 202 Fat 4.8 g Carbs 1.7 g Protein 35.9 g

Glazed Pork Tenderloin

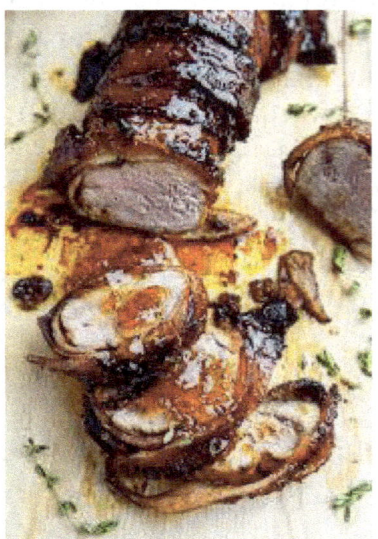

Basic Recipe
Preparation Time: 15 minutes
Cooking Time: 20 minutes
Servings: 3
Ingredients:

- 1-pound pork tenderloin
- 2 tablespoons Sriracha
- 2 tablespoons honey
- Salt, as required

Directions:

1. Insert the rotisserie rod through the pork tenderloin.
2. Insert the rotisserie forks, one on each side of the rod to secure the pork tenderloin.
3. In a small bowl, add the Sriracha, honey and salt and mix well.

4. Brush the pork tenderloin with honey mixture evenly.
5. Arrange the drip pan in the bottom of Instant Vortex Plus Air Fryer Oven cooking chamber.
6. Select "Air Fry" and then adjust the temperature to 350 degrees F.
7. Set the timer for 20 minutes and press the "Start".
8. When the display shows "Add Food" press the red lever down and load the left side of the rod into the Vortex.
9. Now, slide the rod's left side into the groove along the metal bar so it doesn't move.
10. Then, close the door and touch "Rotate".
11. Press the red lever to release the rod when cooking time is complete.
12. Remove the pork from Vortex and place onto a platter for about 10 minutes before slicing.
13. With a sharp knife, cut the roast into desired sized slices and serve.

Nutrition: Calories 269 Fat 5.3 g Carbs 13.5 g Protein 39.7 g

Country Style Pork Tenderloin

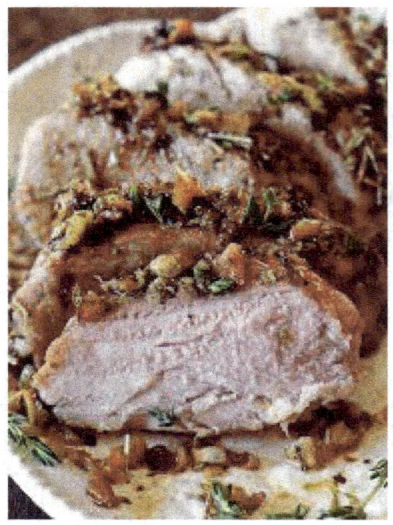

Basic Recipe
Preparation Time: 15 minutes
Cooking Time: 25 minutes
Servings: 3

Ingredients:

- 1-pound pork tenderloin
- 1 tablespoon garlic, minced
- 2 tablespoons soy sauce
- 2 tablespoons honey
- 1 tablespoon Dijon mustard
- 1 tablespoon grain mustard
- 1 teaspoon Sriracha sauce

Directions:

1. In a large bowl, add all the ingredients except pork and mix well.
2. Add the pork tenderloin and coat with the mixture generously.
3. Refrigerate to marinate for 2-3 hours.

---

4. Remove the pork tenderloin from bowl, reserving the marinade.
5. Place the pork tenderloin onto the lightly greased cooking tray.
6. Arrange the drip pan in the bottom of Instant Vortex Plus Air Fryer Oven cooking chamber.
7. Select "Air Fry" and then adjust the temperature to 380 degrees F.
8. Set the timer for 25 minutes and press the ' Start".
9. When the display shows "Add Food" insert the cooking tray in the center position.
10. When the display shows "Turn Food" turn the pork and oat with the reserved marinade.
11. When cooking time is complete, remove the tray from Vortex and place the pork tenderloin onto a platter for about 10 minutes before slicing.
12. With a sharp knife, cut the pork tenderloin into desired sized slices and serve.

Nutrition: Calories 277 Fat 5.7 g Carbs 14.2 g Protein 40.7 g

Seasoned Pork Chops

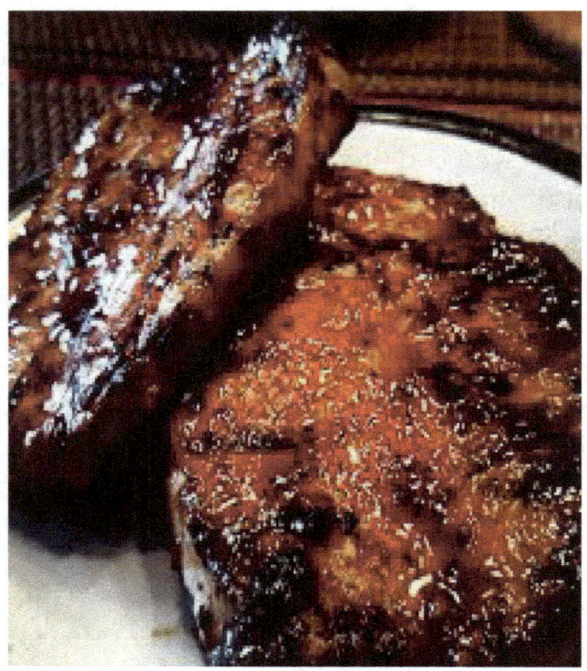

Basic Recipe
Preparation Time: 10 minutes
Cooking Time: 12 minutes
Servings: 4

Ingredients:

- 4 (6-ounce) boneless pork chops
- 2 tablespoons pork rub
- 1 tablespoon olive oil

Directions:

1. Coat both sides of the pork chops with the oil and then, rub with the pork rub.
2. Place the pork chops onto the lightly greased cooking tray.

3. Arrange the drip pan in the bottom of Instant Vortex Plus Air Fryer Oven cooking chamber.
4. Select "Air Fry" and then adjust the temperature to 400 degrees F.
5. Set the timer for 12 minutes and press the ' Start".
6. When the display shows "Add Food" insert the cooking tray in the center position.
7. When the display shows "Turn Food" turn the pork chops.
8. When cooking time is complete, remove the tray from Vortex and serve hot.

Nutrition: Calories 285 Fat 9.5 g Carbs 1.5 g Protein 44.5 g

Breaded Pork Chops

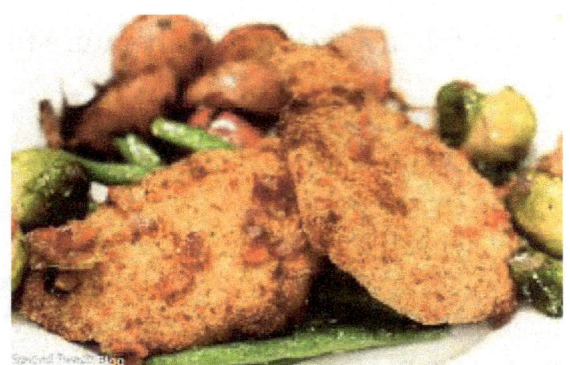

Basic Recipe
Preparation Time: 15 minutes
Cooking Time: 28 minutes
Servings: 2

Ingredients:

- 2 (5-ounce) boneless pork chops
- 1 cup buttermilk
- ½ cup flour
- 1 teaspoon garlic powder
- Salt and ground black pepper, as required
- Olive oil cooking spray

Directions:

1. In a bowl, place the chops and buttermilk and refrigerate, covered for about 12 hours.
2. Remove the chops from the bowl of buttermilk, discarding the buttermilk.
3. In a shallow dish, mix together the flour, garlic powder, salt, and black pepper.
4. Coat the chops with flour mixture generously.
5. Place the pork chops onto the cooking tray and spray with the cooking spray.

6. Arrange the drip pan in the bottom of Instant Vortex Plus Air Fryer Oven cooking chamber.
7. Select "Air Fry" and then adjust the temperature to 380 degrees F.
8. Set the timer for 28 minutes and press the "Start".
9. When the display shows "Add Food" insert the cooking tray in the center position.
10. When the display shows "Turn Food" turn the pork chops.
11. When cooking time is complete, remove the tray from Vortex and serve hot.

Nutrition: Calories 370 Fat 6.4 g Carbs 30.7 g Protein 44.6 g

Crusted Rack of Lamb

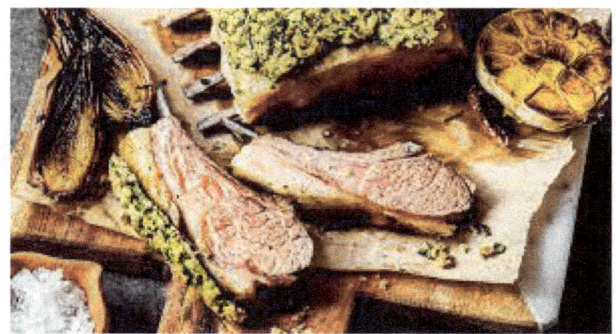

Intermediate Recipe
Preparation Time: 15 minutes
Cooking Time: 19 minutes
Servings: 4

Ingredients:

- 1 rack of lamb, trimmed all fat and frenched
- Salt and ground black pepper, as required
- 1/3 cup pistachios, chopped finely
- 2 tablespoons panko breadcrumbs
- 2 teaspoons fresh thyme, chopped finely
- 1 teaspoon fresh rosemary, chopped finely
- 1 tablespoon butter, melted
- 1 tablespoon Dijon mustard

Directions:

1. Insert the rotisserie rod through the rack on the meaty side of the ribs, right next to the bone.
2. Insert the rotisserie forks, one on each side of the rod to secure the rack.
3. Season the rack with salt and black pepper evenly.
4. Arrange the drip pan in the bottom of Instant Vortex Plus Air Fryer Oven cooking chamber.

5. Select "Air Fry" and then adjust the temperature to 380 degrees F.
6. Set the timer for 12 minutes and press the "Start".
7. When the display shows "Add Food" press the red lever down and load the left side of the rod into the Vortex.
8. Now, slide the rod's left side into the groove along the metal bar so it doesn't move.
9. Then, close the door and touch "Rotate".
10. Meanwhile, in a small bowl, mix together the remaining ingredients except the mustard.
11. Press the red lever to release the rod when cooking time is complete..
12. Remove the rack from Vortex and brush the meaty side with the mustard.
13. Then, coat the pistachio mixture on all sides of the rack and press firmly.
14. Now, place the rack of lamb onto the cooking tray, meat side up.
15. Select "Air Fry" and adjust the temperature to 380 degrees F.
16. Set the timer for 7 minutes and press the "Start".
17. When the display shows "Add Food" insert the cooking tray in the center position.
18. When the display shows "Turn Food" do nothing.
19. When cooking time is complete, remove the tray from Vortex and place the rack onto a cutting board for at least 10 minutes
20. Cut the rack into individual chops and serve.

Nutrition: Calories 824 Fat 39.3 g Carbs 10.3 g Protein 72 g

Lamb Burgers

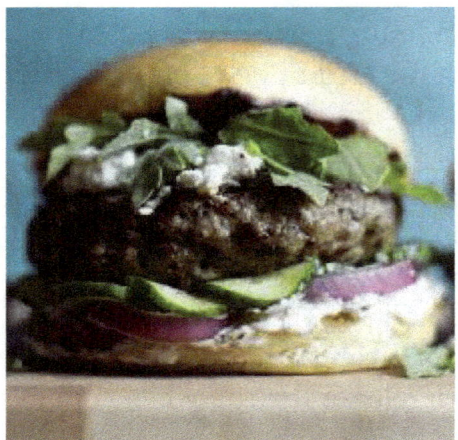

Preparation Time: 15 minutes
Cooking Time: 8 minutes
Servings: 6

Ingredients:

- 2 pounds ground lamb
- 1 tablespoon onion powder
- Salt and ground black pepper, as required

Directions:

1. In a bowl, add all the ingredients and mix well.
2. Make 6 equal-sized patties from the mixture.
3. Arrange the patties onto a cooking tray.
4. Arrange the drip pan in the bottom of Instant Vortex Plus Air Fryer Oven cooking chamber.
5. Select "Air Fry" and then adjust the temperature to 360 degrees F.
6. Set the timer for 8 minutes and press the "Start".
7. When the display shows "Add Food" insert the cooking rack in the center position.

8. When the display shows "Turn Food" turn the burgers.
9. When cooking time is complete, remove the tray from Vortex and serve hot.

Nutrition: Calories 285 Fat 11.1 g Carbs 0.9 g Protein 42.6 g

Salmon

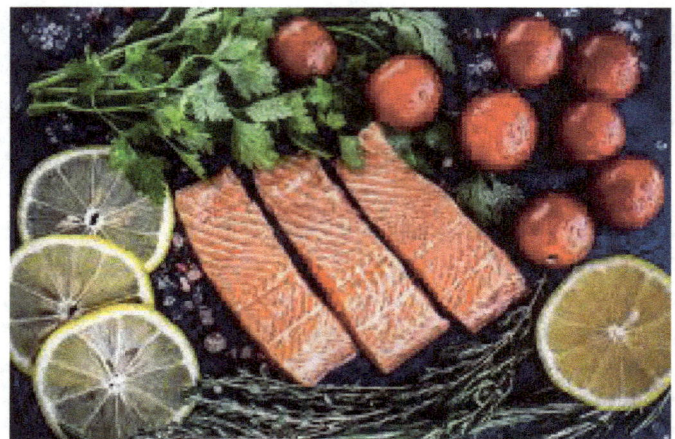

Basic Recipe
Preparation Time: 5 minutes
Cooking Time: 12 minutes
Servings: 2

Ingredients

- 2 salmon fillets, wild-caught, each about 1 ½ inch thick
- 1 teaspoon ground black pepper
- 2 teaspoons paprika
- 1 teaspoon salt
- 2 teaspoons olive oil

Directions:

1. Switch on the air fryer, insert fryer basket, grease it with olive oil, then shut with its lid, set the fryer at 390 degrees F and preheat for 5 minutes. Meanwhile, rub each salmon fillet with oil and then season with black pepper, paprika, and salt.

2. Open the fryer, add seasoned salmon in it, close with its lid and cook for 7 minutes until nicely golden and cooked, flipping the fillets halfway through the

frying. When air fryer beeps, open its lid, transfer salmon onto a serving plate and serve.

Nutrition: Calories 288 Cal Carbs 1.4g Fat 18.9g Protein 28.3g

Parmesan Shrimp

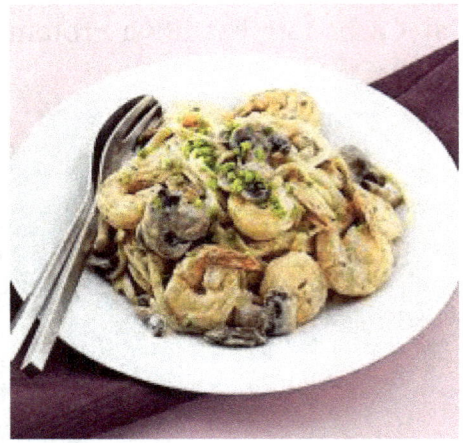

Basic Recipe
Preparation Time: 10 minutes
Cooking Time: 10 minutes
Servings: 6

Ingredients

- 2 pounds jumbo shrimp, wild-caught, peeled, deveined
- 2 tablespoons minced garlic
- 1 teaspoon onion powder
- 1 teaspoon basil
- 1 teaspoon ground black pepper
- 1/2 teaspoon dried oregano
- 2 tablespoons olive oil
- 2/3 cup grated parmesan cheese, reduced Fat
- 2 tablespoons lemon juice

Directions:

1. Switch on the air fryer, insert fryer basket, grease it with olive oil, then shut with its lid, set the fryer at 350 degrees F and preheat for 5 minutes

2. Meanwhile, place cheese in a bowl, add remaining ingredients except for shrimps and lemon juice and stir until combined.
3. Add shrimps and then toss until well coated.
4. Open the fryer, add shrimps in it, spray oil over them, close with its lid and cook for 10 minutes until nicely golden and crispy, shaking halfway through the frying. When air fryer beeps, open its lid, transfer chicken onto a serving plate, Drizzle with lemon juice and serve.

Nutrition: Calories 307 Cal Carbs 12g Fat 16.4g Protein 27.6g

Fish Sticks

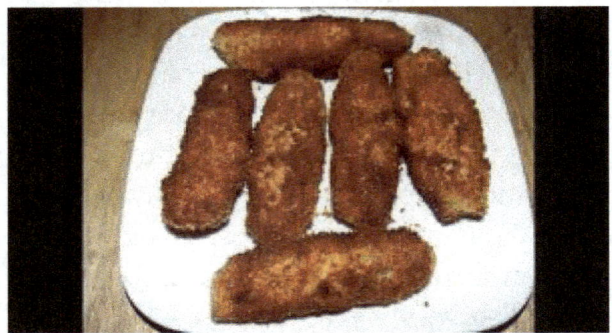

Basic Recipe
Preparation Time: 5 minutes
Cooking Time: 15 minutes
Servings: 4

Ingredients

- 1-pound cod, wild-caught
- ½ teaspoon ground black pepper
- 3/4 teaspoon Cajun seasoning
- 1 teaspoon salt
- 1 1/2 cups pork rind
- 1/4 cup mayonnaise, reduced Fat
- 2 tablespoons water
- 2 tablespoons Dijon mustard

Directions:

1. Switch on the air fryer, insert fryer basket, grease it with olive oil, then shut with its lid, set the fryer at 400 degrees F and preheat for 5 minutes
2. Meanwhile, place mayonnaise in a bowl and then whisk in water and mustard until blended.
3. Place pork rinds in a shallow dish, add Cajun seasoning, black pepper and salt and stir until mixed.

4. Cut the cod into 1 by 2 inches pieces, then dip into mayonnaise mixture and then coat with pork rind mixture.
5. Open the fryer; add fish sticks in it, spray with oil, close with its lid and cook for 10 minutes until nicely golden and crispy, flipping the sticks halfway through the frying.
6. When air fryer beeps, open its lid, transfer fish sticks onto a serving plate and serve.

Nutrition: Calories 263 Cal Carbs 1g Fat 16g Protein 26.4g

Shrimp with Lemon and Chile

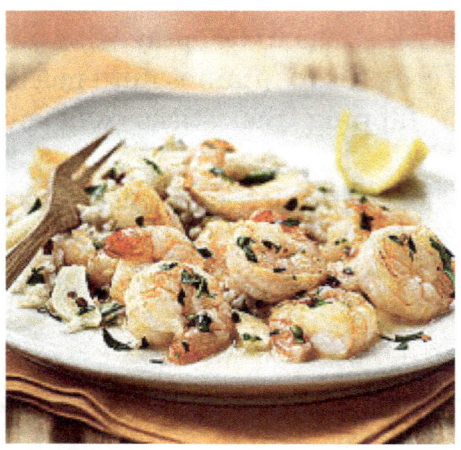

Basic Recipe
Preparation Time: 5 minutes
Cooking Time: 12 minutes
Servings: 2

Ingredients:

- 1-pound shrimp, wild-caught, peeled, deveined
- 1 lemon, sliced
- 1 small red chili pepper, sliced
- ½ teaspoon ground black pepper
- 1/2 teaspoon garlic powder
- 1 teaspoon salt
- 1 tablespoon olive oil

Directions:

1. Switch on the air fryer, insert fryer basket, grease it with olive oil, then shut with its lid, set the fryer at 400 degrees F and preheat for 5 minutes

2. Meanwhile, place shrimps in a bowl, add garlic, salt, black pepper, oil, and lemon slices and toss until combined.Open the fryer, add shrimps and lemon in it close with its lid and cook for 5 minutes, shaking halfway through the frying. Then add chili slices, shake the basket until mixed and continue cooking for 2 minutes or until shrimps are opaque and crispy. When air fryer beeps, open its lid, transfer shrimps and lemon slices onto a serving plate and serve.

Nutrition: Calories 112.5 Cal Carbs 1g Fat 1g   Protein 2g

Tilapia

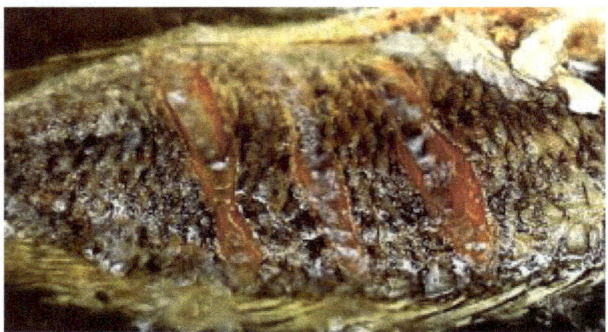

Basic Recipe
Preparation Time: 5 minutes
Cooking Time: 12 minutes
Servings: 2

Ingredients:

- 2 tilapia fillets, wild-caught, 1 ½ inch thick
- 1 teaspoon old bay seasoning
- ¾ teaspoon lemon pepper seasoning
- ½ teaspoon salt

Directions:

1. Switch on the air fryer, insert fryer basket, grease it with olive oil, then shut with its lid, set the fryer at 400 degrees F and preheat for 5 minutes
2. Meanwhile, spray tilapia fillets with oil and then season with salt, lemon pepper, and old bay seasoning until evenly coated.Open the fryer, add tilapia in it, close with its lid and cook for 7 minutes until nicely golden and cooked, turning the fillets halfway through the frying.When air fryer beeps, open its lid, transfer tilapia fillets onto a serving plate and serve.

Nutrition: Calories 36 Cal Carbs 0g Fat 0.75g Protein 7.4g

Tomato Basil Scallops

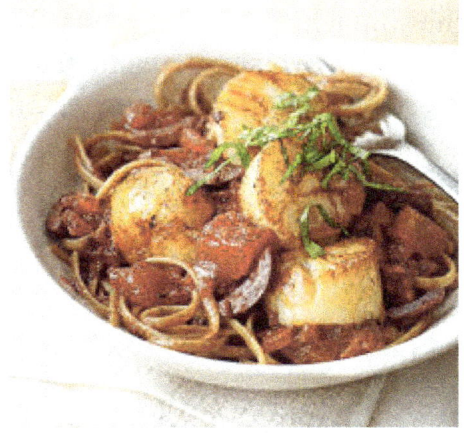

Basic Recipe
Preparation Time: 5 minutes
Cooking Time: 15 minutes
Servings: 2

Ingredients:

- 8 jumbo sea scallops, wild-caught
- 1 tablespoon tomato paste
- 12 ounces frozen spinach, thawed and dry outed
- 1 tablespoon chopped fresh basil
- 1 teaspoon ground black pepper
- 1 teaspoon minced garlic
- 1 teaspoon salt
- 3/4 cup heavy whipping cream, reduced Fat

Directions:

1. Switch on the air fryer, insert fryer basket, grease it with olive oil, then shut with its lid, set the fryer at 350 degrees F and preheat for 5 minutes
2. Meanwhile, take a 7 inches baking pan, grease it with oil and place spinach in it in an even layer.

3. Spray the scallops with oil, sprinkle with ½ teaspoon each of salt and black pepper and then place scallops over the spinach.
4. Place tomato paste in a bowl, whisk in cream, basil, garlic, and remaining salt and black pepper until smooth, and then pour over the scallops.
5. Open the fryer, place the pan in it, close with its lid and cook for 10 minutes until thoroughly cooked and sauce is hot.
6. Serve straight away.

Nutrition: Calories 359 Cal Carbs 6g Fat 33g Protein 9g

Shrimp Scampi

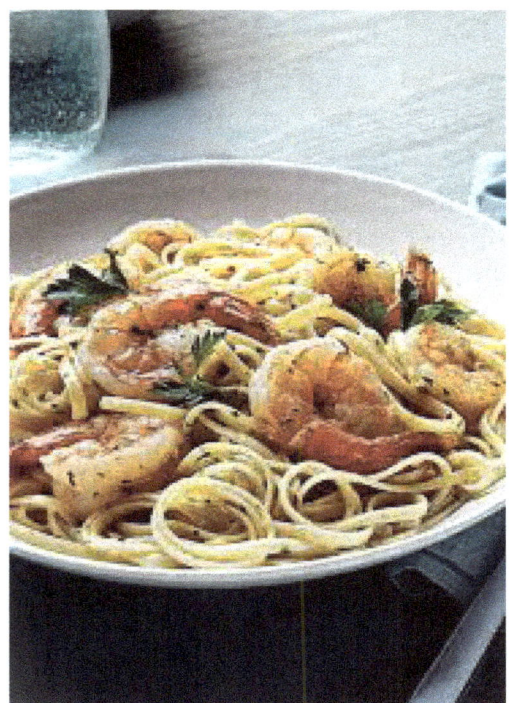

Basic Recipe
Preparation Time: 5 minutes
Cooking Time: 12 minutes
Servings: 4
Ingredients:

- 1-pound shrimp, peeled, deveined
- 1 tablespoon minced garlic
- 1 tablespoon minced basil
- 1 tablespoon lemon juice
- 1 teaspoon dried chives
- 1 teaspoon dried basil
- 2 teaspoons red pepper flakes
- 4 tablespoons butter, unsalted

- 2 tablespoons chicken stock

Directions:

1. Switch on the air fryer, insert fryer pan, grease it with olive oil, then shut with its lid, set the fryer at 330 degrees F and preheat for 5 minutes
2. Add butter in it along with red pepper and garlic and cook for 2 minutes or until the butter has melted.
3. Then add remaining ingredients in the pan, stir until mixed and continue cooking for 5 minutes until shrimps have cooked, stirring halfway through.
4. When done, remove the pan from the air fryer, stir the shrimp scampi, let it rest for 1 minute and then stir again.
5. Garnish shrimps with basil leaves and serve.

Nutrition: Calories 221 Cal Carbs 1g Fat 13g Protein 23g

Salmon Cakes

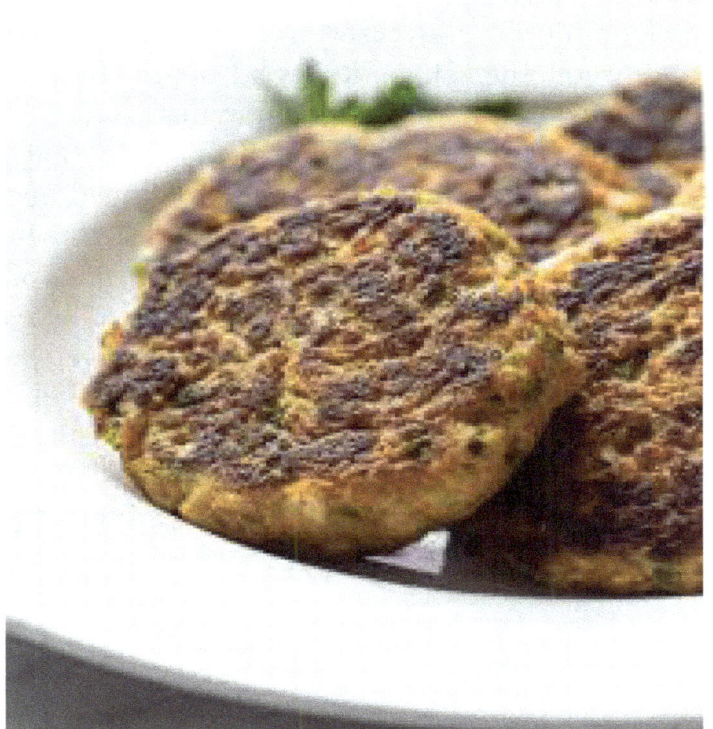

Basic Recipe
Preparation Time: 5 minutes
Cooking Time: 12 minutes
Servings: 2
Ingredients:
- ½ cup almond flour
- 15 ounces cooked pink salmon
- ¼ teaspoon ground black pepper
- 2 teaspoons Dijon mustard
- 2 tablespoons chopped fresh dill

———

- 2 tablespoons mayonnaise, reduced Fat
- 1 egg, pastured
- 2 wedges of lemon

Directions:

1. Switch on the air fryer, insert fryer basket, grease it with olive oil, then shut with its lid, set the fryer at 400 degrees F and preheat for 5 minutes

2. Meanwhile, place all the ingredients in a bowl, except for lemon wedges, stir until combined and then shape into four patties, each about 4-inches. Open the fryer, add salmon patties in it, spray oil over them, close with its lid and cook for 12 minutes until nicely golden and crispy, flipping the patties halfway through the frying.

3. When air fryer beeps, open its lid, transfer salmon patties onto a serving plate and serve.

Nutrition: Calories 517 Cal Carbs 15g Fat 27g Protein 52g

Cilantro Lime Shrimps

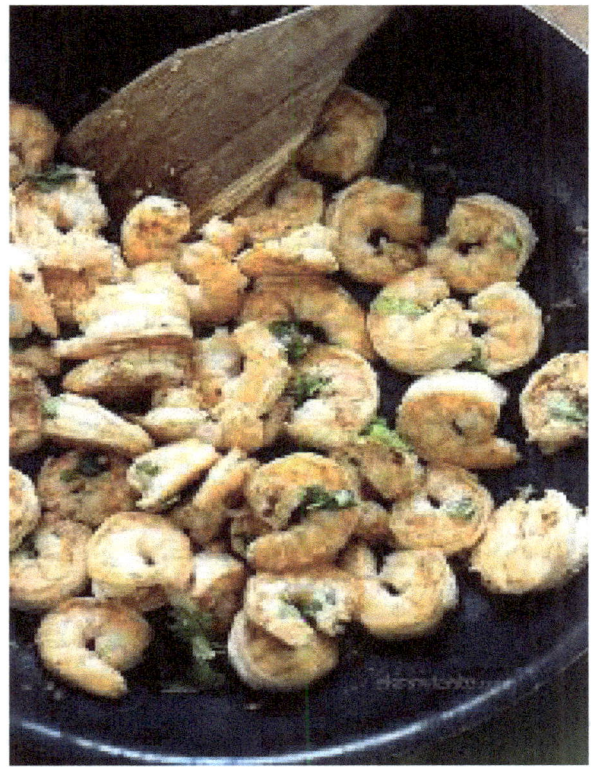

Basic Recipe
Preparation Time: 25 minutes
Cooking Time: 21 minutes
Servings: 4

Ingredients:

- 1/2-pound shrimp, peeled, deveined
- 1/2 teaspoon minced garlic
- 1 tablespoon chopped cilantro
- 1/2 teaspoon paprika
- ¾ teaspoon salt
- 1/2 teaspoon ground cumin
- 2 tablespoons lemon juice

Directions:

1. Take 6 wooden skewers and let them soak in warm water for 20 minutes
2. Meanwhile, switch on the air fryer, insert fryer basket, grease it with olive oil, then shut with its lid, set the fryer at 350 degrees F and let preheat.
3. Whisk together lemon juice, paprika, salt, cumin, and garlic in a large bowl, then add shrimps and toss until well coated.
4. Dry out the skewers and then thread shrimps in them.
5. Open the fryer, add shrimps in it in a single layer, spray oil over them, close with its lid and cook for 8 minutes until nicely golden and cooked, turning the skewers halfway through the frying.
6. When air fryer beeps, open its lid, transfer shrimps onto a serving plate and keep them warm.
7. Cook remaining shrimp skewers in the same manner and serve.

Nutrition: Calories 59 Cal Carbs 0.3g Fat 1.5g Protein 11g

Cajun Style Shrimp

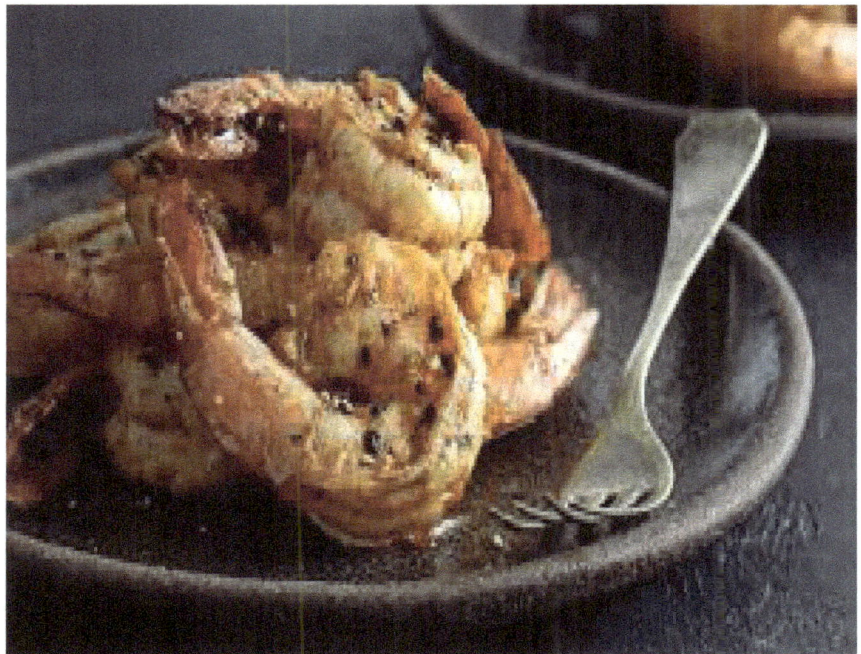

Basic Recipe
Preparation Time: 3 minutes
Cooking Time: 10 minutes
Servings: 2
Ingredients:
- 6g of salt
- 2g smoked paprika
- 2ggarlic powder
- 2g Italian seasoning
- 2g chili powder
- 1g onion powder
- 1g cayenne pepper
- 1g black pepper
- 1g dried thyme

- 454g large shrimp, peeled and unveiled
- 30 ml of olive oil
- Lime wedges, to serve

Directions:

1. Select Preheat, in the air fryer, set the temperature to 190°C and press Start/Pause.Combine all seasonings in a large bowl. Set aside
2. Mix the shrimp with olive oil until they are evenly coated. Sprinkle the dressing mixture over the shrimp and stir until well coated. Place the shrimp in the preheated air fryer.
3. Select Shrimp set the time to 5 minutes and press Start/Pause. Shake the baskets in the middle of cooking. Serve with pieces of lime.

Nutrition: Calories 126 Fat 6g Carbs 2g Proteins: 33g

Crab Cakes

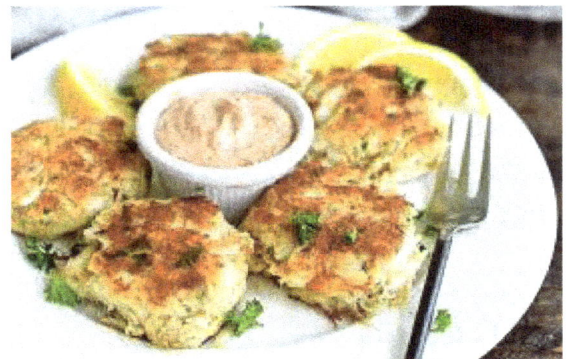

Intermediate Recipe
Preparation Time: 10 minutes
Cooking Time: 40 minutes
Servings: 2
Ingredients:

- For crab cakes:
- 1 large egg, beaten
- 17g of mayonnaise
- 11g Dijon mustard
- 5 ml Worcestershire sauce
- 2g Old Bay seasoning
- 2g of salt
- A pinch of white pepper
- A pinch of cayenne
- 26g celery, finely diced
- 45g red pepper, finely diced
- 8g fresh parsley, finely chopped
- 227g of crab meat
- 28g breadcrumbs
- Nonstick Spray Oil
- Remodeled:

- 55g of mayonnaise
- 15g capers washed and dry outed
- 5g sweet pickles, chopped
- 5g red onion, finely chopped
- 8 ml of lemon juice
- 8g Dijon mustard
- Salt and pepper to taste

Directions:

1. Mix the ingredients of remodeled until everything is well incorporated. Set aside
2. Beat the egg, mayonnaise, mustard, Worcestershire sauce, Old Bay seasoning, salt, white pepper, cayenne pepper, celery, pepper, and parsley.
3. Gently stir the crab meat in the egg mixture and stir it until well mixed.Sprinkle the breadcrumbs over the crab mixture and fold them gently until the breadcrumbs cover every corner.
4. Shape the crab mixture into 4 cakes and chill in the fridge for 30 minutes. Select Preheat in the air fryer and press Start/Pause.
5. Place a sheet of baking paper in the basket of the preheated air fryer. Sprinkle the crab cakes with cooking spray and place them gently on the paper.Cook the crab cakes at 205°C for 8 minutes until golden brown.
6. Flip crab cakes during cooking. Serve with remodeled.

Nutrition: Calories 110 Fat 6.5g Carbs 5.5g Protein 7g

Tuna Pie

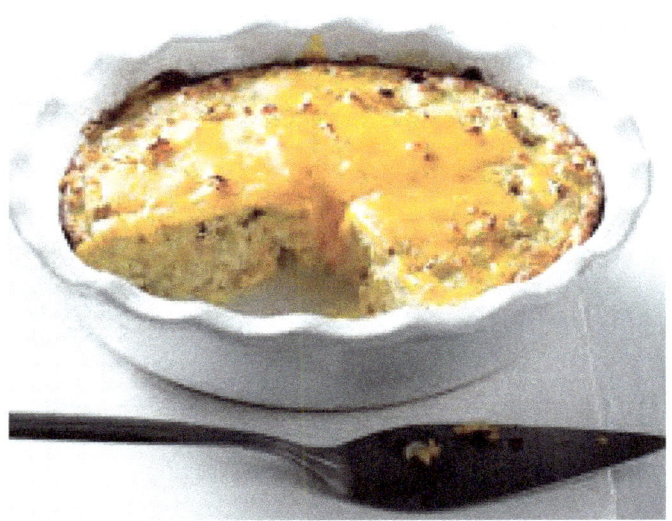

Basic Recipe
Preparation Time: 10 minutes
Cooking Time: 30 minutes
Serving: 4

Ingredients:

- 2 hard-boiled eggs
- 2 tuna cans
- 200 ml fried tomato
- 1 sheet of broken dough

Directions:

1. Cut the eggs into small pieces and mix with the tuna and tomato.
2. Spread the sheet of broken dough and cut into two equal squares.

3. Put the mixture of tuna, eggs, and tomato on one of the squares.
4. Cover with the other, join at the ends and decorate with leftover little pieces.
5. Preheat the air fryer a few minutes at 180oC.
6. Enter in the air fryer basket and set the timer for 15 minutes at 180oC

Nutrition: Calories 244 Fat 13.67g Carbs 21.06g Protein 8.72g

Tuna Puff Pastry

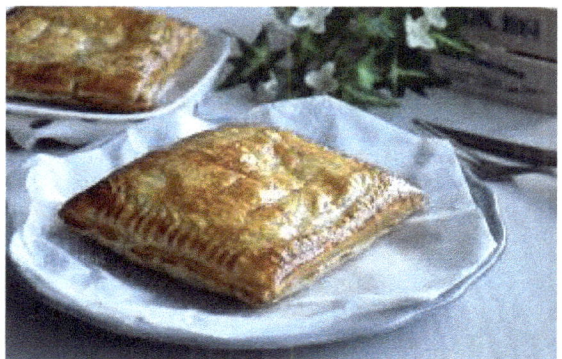

Basic Recipe
Preparation Time: 5 minutes
Cooking Time: 15 minutes
Serving: 2

Ingredients:

- 2 square puff pastry dough, bought ready
- 1 egg (white and yolk separated)
- ½ cup tuna tea
- ½ cup chopped parsley tea
- ½ cup chopped tea olives
- Salt and pepper to taste

Directions:

1. Preheat the air fryer. Set the timer of 5 minutes and the temperature to 200C.
2. Mix the tuna with olives and parsley. Season to taste and set aside. Place half of the filling each dough and fold in half. Brush with egg white and close gently. After closing, make two small cuts at the top of the air outlet. Brush with the egg yolk.
3. Place in the basket of the air fryer. Set the time to 10 minutes and press the power button.

Nutrition: Calories 291 Fat 16g Carbs 26g Protein 8g

Cajun Style Catfish

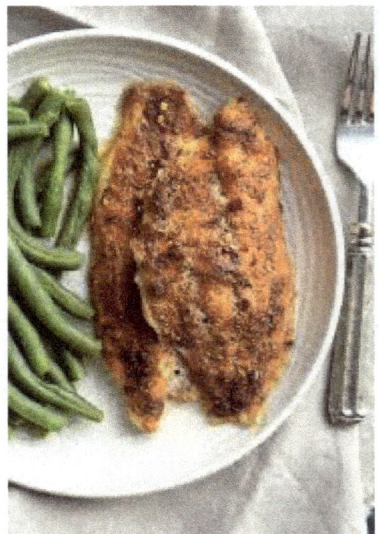

Basic Recipe
Preparation Time: 3 minutes
Cooking Time: 7 minutes
Servings: 2

Ingredients:

- 5g of paprika
- 3ggarlic powder
- 2g onion powder
- 2gground dried thyme
- 1gground black pepper
- 1g cayenne pepper
- 1g dried basil
- 1g dried oregano
- 2 catfish fillets (6 oz)
- Nonstick Spray Oil

Directions:

1. Preheat the air fryer for a few minutes. Set the temperature to 175°C.
2. Mix all seasonings in a bowl. Cover the fish generously on each side with the dressing mixture.
3. Spray each side of the fish with oil spray and place it in the preheated air fryer.
4. Select Marine Food and press Start /Pause.
5. Remove carefully when you finish cooking and serve on semolina.

Nutrition: Calories 228 Fat; 13g Carbs 0g Protein 20g

Tuna Chipotle

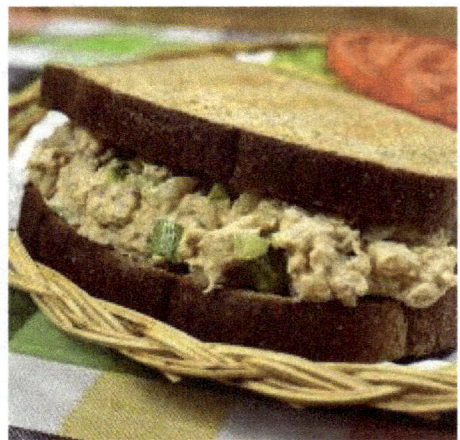

Basic Recipe
Preparation Time: 5 minutes
Cooking Time: 8 minutes
Servings: 2

Ingredients:

- 142g tuna
- 45g chipotle sauce
- 4 slices of white bread
- 2 slices of pepper jack cheese

Directions:

1. Preheat the air fryer set the temperature to 160°C. Mix the tuna and chipotle until combined.
2. Spread half of the chipotle tuna mixture on each of the 2 slices of bread.
3. Add a slice of pepper jack cheese on each and close with the remaining 2 slices of bread, making 2 sandwiches.
4. Place the sandwiches in the preheated air fryer. Set the timer to 8 minutes
5. Cut diagonally and serve.

Nutrition:
Calories 121 Fat 4g Carbs 2g Protein 16g

Fish Tacos

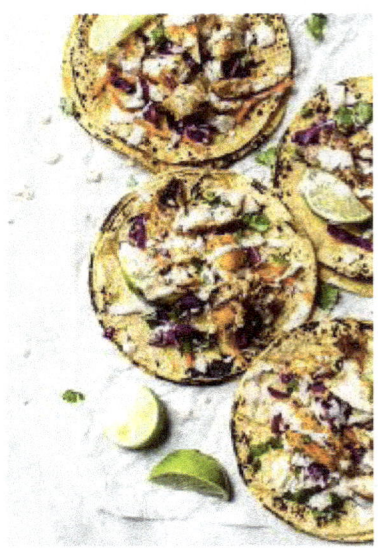

Basic Recipe
Preparation Time: 10 minutes
Cooking Time: 7 minutes
Servings: 4-5
Ingredients:
- 454g of tilapia, cut into strips of
- 38 mm thick
- 52g yellow cornmeal
- 1gground cumin
- 1g chili powder
- 2ggarlic powder
- 1g onion powder
- 3g of salt
- 1g black pepper
- Nonstick Spray Oil
- Corn tortillas, to serve
- Tartar sauce, to serve

- Lime wedges, to serve

Directions:

1. Cut the tilapia into strips 38 mm thick.
2. Mix cornmeal and seasonings in a shallow dish.
3. Cover the fish strips with seasoned cornmeal. Set aside in the fridge.
4. Preheat the air fryer for 5 minutes
5. Set the temperature to 170°C.
6. Sprinkle the fish coated with oil spray and place it in the preheated air fryer.
7. Put the fish in the air fryer, set the timer to 7 minutes
8. Turn the fish halfway through cooking.
9. Serve the fish in corn tortillas with tartar sauce and a splash of lemon.

Nutrition: Calories 108 Fat 26g Carbs 11g Protein 9g

Tomato Soup

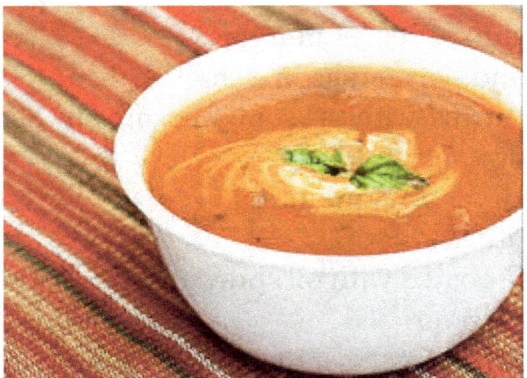

Basic Recipe
Preparation Time: 10 minutes
Cooking Time: 7 minutes
Servings: 4

Ingredients:

- 2 tablespoons of homemade tomato sauce
- 2 teaspoons of dried basil, crushed
- 4 cups of low-sodium vegetable broth
- 1 tablespoon of balsamic vinegar
- 3 pounds of fresh tomatoes, chopped
- 1 tablespoon of olive oil
- 2 teaspoons of dried parsley, crushed
- 2 tablespoons of sugar
- 1 medium onion, chopped
- Freshly ground black pepper, to taste
- ¼ cup of fresh basil, chopped
- 1 garlic clove, minced

Directions:

1. Set the Instant Vortex on Air fryer to 365 degrees F for 5 minutes

2. Put the tomatoes, garlic, onion, and fresh basil in the cooking tray.
3. Insert the cooking tray in the Vortex when it displays "Add Food". Remove from the Vortex when cooking time is complete.
4. Put the olive oil in a wok and add the tomatoes mixture, tomato sauce, dried herbs, broth, and black pepper.
5. Secure the lid of the wok and cook for about 12 minutes on medium heat.
6. Fold in the sugar and vinegar.
7. Pour into the immersion blender and puree the soup to serve hot.

Nutrition: Calories 146   Fat 4.5gCarbs 23.5gProtein 5.4g

Roasted Tomatoes

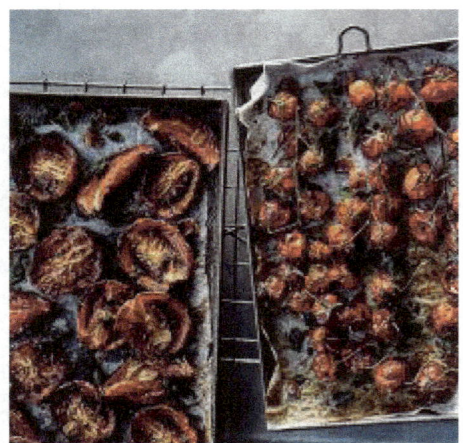

Basic Recipe
Preparation Time: 5 minutes
Cooking Time: 8 minutes
Servings: 4

Ingredients:

- 1 tablespoon of herbed butter
- 4 large tomatoes
- 1 cup of mozzarella cheese, shredded

Directions:

1. Set the Instant Vortex on Roast to 365 degrees F for 10 minutes Scoop out the internal filling of the tomatoes and stuff with the cheese.
2. Place the stuffed tomatoes on the cooking tray and top with the herbed butter. Insert the cooking tray in the Vortex when it displays "Add Food". Remove from the Vortex when cooking time is complete. Serve warm.

Nutrition: Calories 75 Fat 3.2g Carbs 7.5g Protein 5g

Bacon Potato Cheesy Soup

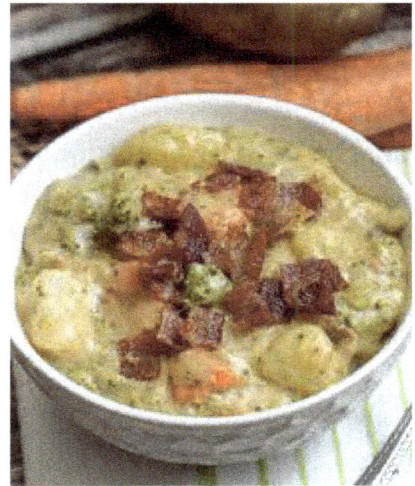

Basic Recipe
Preparation Time: 5 minutes
Cooking Time: 20 minutes
Servings: 4
Ingredients:

- 1 cup of cheddar cheese, shredded
- 1 cup of frozen corn
- 3 tablespoons of butter
- ¼ teaspoon of red paprika flakes
- 8 large potatoes, peeled and cubed
- 1 teaspoon of salt
- 2 cups of half and half cream
- 1 teaspoon of black pepper
- 2 tablespoons of dried parsley
- 3 oz. of cream cheese, cubed
- 6 slices bacon, crumbled
- ½ cup of onions, chopped
- 3 cups of chicken broth

—

Directions:
1. Set the Instant Vortex on Air fryer to 375 degrees F for 5 minutes Put the potatoes, corn, and bacon in the cooking tray.
2. Insert the cooking tray in the Vortex when it displays "Add Food". Remove from the Vortex when cooking time is complete.
3. Put the butter in a wok and add the onions. Sauté for about 3 minutes and fold in the potato's mixture with rest of the ingredients.
4. Secure the lid of the wok and cook for about 12 minutes on medium heat.
5. Dish out the potatoes, mash them well and return to the pot.
6. Stir the soup well and serve hot.

Nutrition: Calories 669 Protein 20 g Carbs 88g Fat 28g

Bacon and Cauliflower Soup

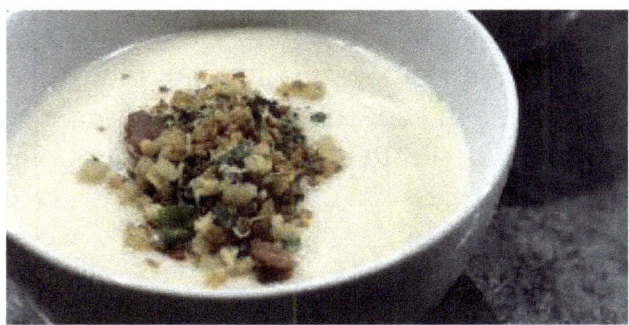

Basic Recipe
Preparation Time: 10 minutes
Cooking Time: 20 minutes
Servings: 4

Ingredients:

- 2 tablespoons of butter
- 4 cups of chicken stock
- 1 large onion, chopped
- 4 potatoes, chopped
- 3 cups of cauliflower florets
- ½ cup of heavy cream
- 1 tablespoon of salt
- 1 tablespoon of black pepper
- 12 slices of bacon, crisp fried

Directions:

1. Set the Instant Vortex on Air fryer to 375 degrees F for 5 minutes Put the bacon, potatoes, and cauliflower in the cooking tray. Insert the cooking tray in the Vortex when it displays "Add Food". Remove from the Vortex when cooking time is complete. Put the butter in a wok and add the onions.

2. Sauté it for about 3 minutes and then stirs in the bacon mixture and the chicken stock. Secure the lid of the wok and cook for about 10 minutes on medium heat. Pour this mixture into an immersion blender and puree it. Ladle out in a bowl to serve.

Nutrition: Calories 344 Protein 8.3g Carbs 44.1g Fat 16.7g

DINNER

Thyme Turkey Breast

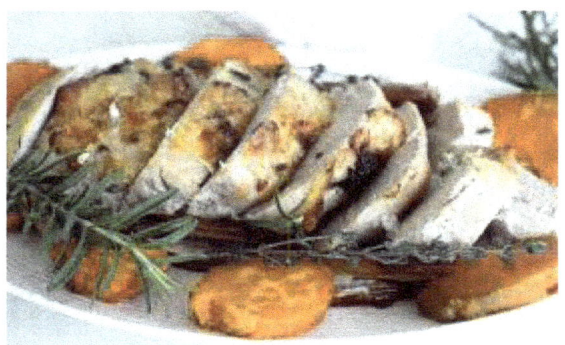

Preparation Time: 10 minutes
Cooking Time: 40 minutes
Serving: 4

Ingredients:
- 2 lb. turkey breast
- Salt, to taste
- Black pepper, to taste
- 4 tablespoon butter, melted
- 3 cloves garlic, minced
- 1 teaspoon thyme, chopped
- 1 teaspoon rosemary, chopped

Directions:
1. Mix butter with salt, black pepper, garlic, thyme, and rosemary in a bowl.
2. Rub this seasoning over the turkey breast liberally and place in the Air Fryer basket.
3. Turn the dial to select the "Air Fry" mode.

---

4. Hit the Time button and again use the dial to set the cooking time to 40 minutes
5. Now push the Temp button and rotate the dial to set the temperature at 375 degrees F.
6. Once preheated, place the Air fryer basket inside the oven
7. Slice and serve fresh.

Nutrition: Calories 334 Fat 4.7 g Carbs 54.1 g Protein 26.2 g

Chicken Drumsticks

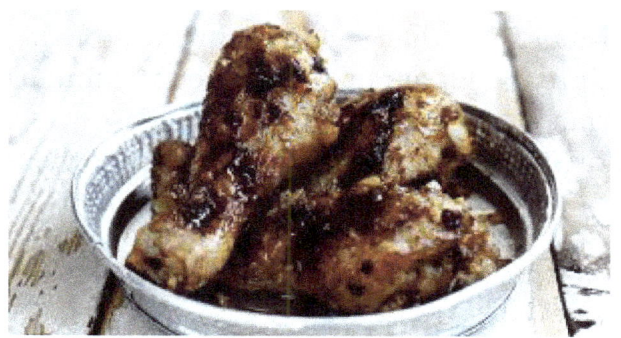

Basic Recipe
Preparation Time: 10 minutes
Cooking Time: 20 minutes
Serving: 8

Ingredients:

- 8 chicken drumsticks
- 2 tablespoon olive oil
- 1 teaspoon salt
- 1 teaspoon pepper
- 1 teaspoon garlic powder
- 1 teaspoon paprika
- 1/2 teaspoon cumin

Directions:

1. Mix olive oil with salt, black pepper, garlic powder, paprika, and cumin in a bowl.
2. Rub this mixture liberally over all the drumsticks.
3. Place these drumsticks in the Air fryer basket.
4. Turn the dial to select the "Air Fry" mode.
5. Hit the Time button and again use the dial to set the cooking time to 20 minutes
6. Now push the Temp button and rotate the dial to set the temperature at 375 degrees F.

7. Once preheated, place the Air fryer basket inside the oven.
8. Flip the drumsticks when cooked halfway through.
9. Resume air frying for another rest of the 10 minutes
10. Serve warm.

Nutrition: Calories 212 Fat 11.8 g Carbs 14.6 g Protein 17.3 g

Blackened Chicken Bake

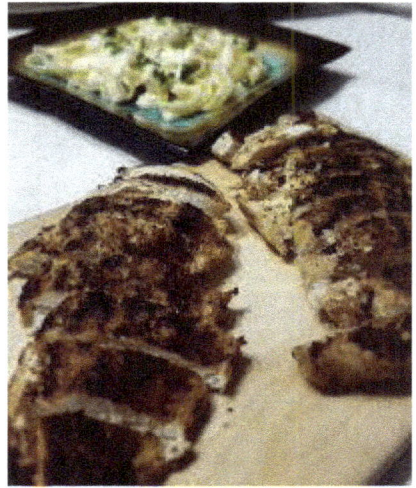

Basic Recipe
Preparation Time: 10 minutes
Cooking Time: 18 minutes
Serving: 4

Ingredients:
- 4 chicken breasts
- 2 teaspoon olive oil
- Seasoning:
- 1 1/2 tablespoon brown sugar
- 1 teaspoon paprika
- 1 teaspoon dried oregano
- 1/4 teaspoon garlic powder
- 1/2 teaspoon salt and pepper
- Garnish:
- Chopped parsley

Directions:
1. Mix olive oil with brown sugar, paprika, oregano, garlic powder, salt, and black pepper in a bowl.

---

2. Place the chicken breasts in the baking tray of the Ninja Oven.
3. Pour and rub this mixture liberally over all the chicken breasts.
4. Turn the dial to select the "Bake" mode.
5. Hit the Time button and again use the dial to set the cooking time to 18 minutes
6. Now push the Temp button and rotate the dial to set the temperature at 425 degrees F.
7. Once preheated, place the baking tray inside the oven
8. Serve warm.

Nutrition: Calories 412 Fat 24.8 g Carbs 43.8 g Protein 18.9 g

Crusted Chicken Drumsticks

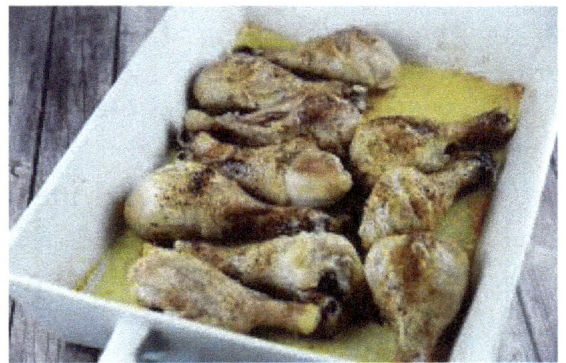

Basic Recipe
Preparation Time: 10 minutes
Cooking Time: 10 minutes
Serving: 4
Ingredients:

- 1 lb. chicken drumsticks
- 1/2 cup buttermilk
- 1/2 cup panko breadcrumbs
- 1/2 cup flour
- 1/4 teaspoon baking powder
- Spice Mixture:
- 1/2 teaspoon salt
- 1/2 teaspoon celery salt
- 1/4 teaspoon oregano
- 1/4 teaspoon cayenne
- 1 teaspoon paprika
- 1/4 teaspoon garlic powder
- 1/4 teaspoon dried thyme
- 1/2 teaspoon ground ginger
- 1/2 teaspoon white pepper
- 1/2 teaspoon black pepper

- 3 tablespoon butter melted

Directions:

1. Soak chicken in the buttermilk and cover to marinate overnight in the refrigerator. Mix spices with flour, breadcrumbs, and baking powder in a shallow tray.
2. Remove the chicken from the milk and coat them well with the flour spice mixture
3. Place the chicken drumsticks in the Air fryer basket of the Ninja Oven.
4. Pour the melted butter over the drumsticks
5. Turn the dial to select the "Air fry" mode. Hit the Time button and again use the dial to set the cooking time to 10 minutes
6. Now push the Temp button and rotate the dial to set the temperature at 425 degrees F.
7. Once preheated, place the baking tray inside the oven
8. Flip the drumsticks and resume cooking for another 10 minutes
9. Serve warm.

Nutrition: Calories 331 Fat 2.5 g Carbs 69 g Protein 28.7g

Brine Soaked Turkey

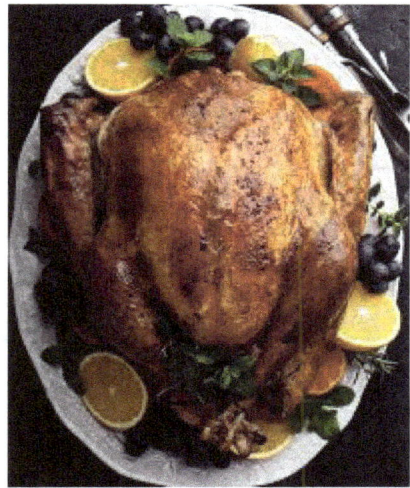

Intermediate Recipe
Preparation Time: 10 minutes
Cooking Time: 45 minutes
Serving: 8
Ingredients:

- 7 lb. bone-in, skin-on turkey breast
- Brine:
- 1/2 cup salt
- 1 lemon
- 1/2 onion
- 3 cloves garlic, smashed
- 5 sprigs fresh thyme
- 3 bay leaves
- Black pepper
- Turkey Breast:
- 4 tablespoon butter, softened
- 1/2 teaspoon black pepper
- 1/2 teaspoon garlic powder

- 1/4 teaspoon dried thyme
- 1/4 teaspoon dried oregano

Directions:

1. Mix the turkey brine ingredients in a pot and soak the turkey in the brine overnight. Next day, remove the soaked turkey from the brine.
2. Whisk the butter, black pepper, garlic powder, oregano, and thyme. Brush the butter mixture over the turkey then place it in a baking tray.
3. Press "Power Button" of Air Fry Oven and turn the dial to select the "Air Roast" mode. Press the Time button and again turn the dial to set the cooking time to 45 minutes
4. Now push the Temp button and rotate the dial to set the temperature at 370 degrees F. Once preheated, place the turkey baking tray in the oven and close its lid.
5. Slice and serve warm.

Nutrition: Calories 397 Fat 15.4 g Carbs 58.5 g Protein 7.9 g

Turkey Meatballs

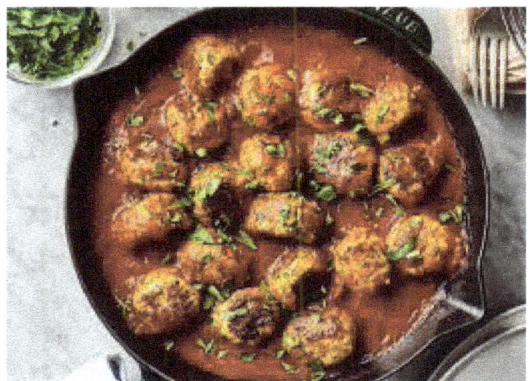

Basic Recipe
Preparation Time: 10 minutes
Cooking Time: 20 minutes
Serving: 6

Ingredients:

- lb. turkey mince
- 1 red bell pepper, deseeded and chopped
- 1 large egg, beaten
- 4 tablespoons parsley, minced
- 1 tablespoon cilantro, minced
- Salt, to taste
- Black pepper, to taste

Directions:

1. Toss all the meatball ingredients in a bowl and mix well. Make small meatballs out this mixture and place them in the air fryer basket.
2. Press "Power Button" of Air Fry Oven and turn the dial to select the "Air Fry" mode. Press the Time button and again turn the dial to set the cooking time to 20 minutes

3. Now push the Temp button and rotate the dial to set the temperature at 375 degrees F.Once preheated, place the air fryer basket inside and close its lid. Serve warm.

Nutrition: Calories 338 Fat 9.7 g Carbs 32.5 g Protein 10.3 g

Ground Chicken Meatballs

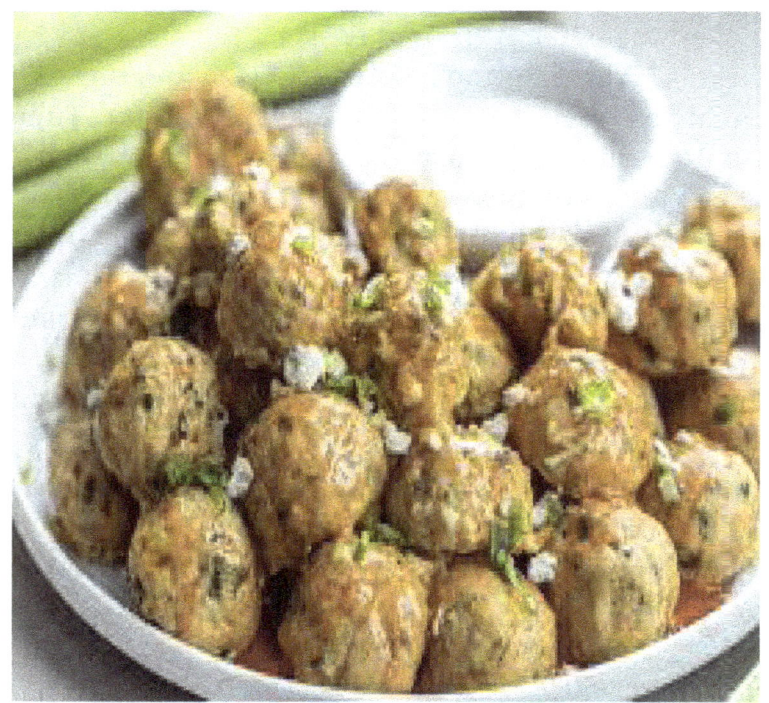

Basic Recipe
Preparation Time: 10 minutes
Cooking Time: 10 minutes
Serving: 4
Ingredients:
- 1-lb. ground chicken
- 1/3 cup panko
- 1 teaspoon salt
- 2 teaspoons chives
- 1/2 teaspoon garlic powder
- 1 teaspoon thyme
- 1 egg

Directions:

1. Toss all the meatball ingredients in a bowl and mix well. Make small meatballs out this mixture and place them in the air fryer basket.
2. Press "Power Button" of Air Fry Oven and turn the dial to select the "Air Fry" mode.Press the Time button and again turn the dial to set the cooking time to 10 minutes
3. Now push the Temp button and rotate the dial to set the temperature at 350 degrees F.Once preheated, place the air fryer basket inside and close its lid. Serve warm.

Nutrition: Calories 453 Fat 2.4 g Carbs 18 g Protein 23.2 g

Parmesan Chicken Meatballs

Basic Recipe
Preparation Time: 10 minutes
Cooking Time: 12 minutes
Serving: 4

Ingredients:
- 1-lb. ground chicken
- 1 large egg, beaten
- ½ cup Parmesan cheese, grated
- ½ cup pork rinds, ground
- 1 teaspoon garlic powder
- 1 teaspoon paprika
- 1 teaspoon kosher salt
- ½ teaspoon pepper
- Crust:
- ½ cup pork rinds, ground

Directions:
1. Toss all the meatball ingredients in a bowl and mix well.Make small meatballs out this mixture and roll them in the pork rinds.
2. Place the coated meatballs in the air fryer basket.Press "Power Button" of Air Fry Oven and turn the dial to select the "Bake" mode.
3. Press the Time button and again turn the dial to set the cooking time to 12 minutes. Now push the Temp button and rotate the dial to set the temperature at 400 degrees F.
4. Once preheated, place the air fryer basket inside and close its lid.
5. Serve warm.

Nutrition:
Calories 529 Fat 17 g Carbs 55 g Protein 41g

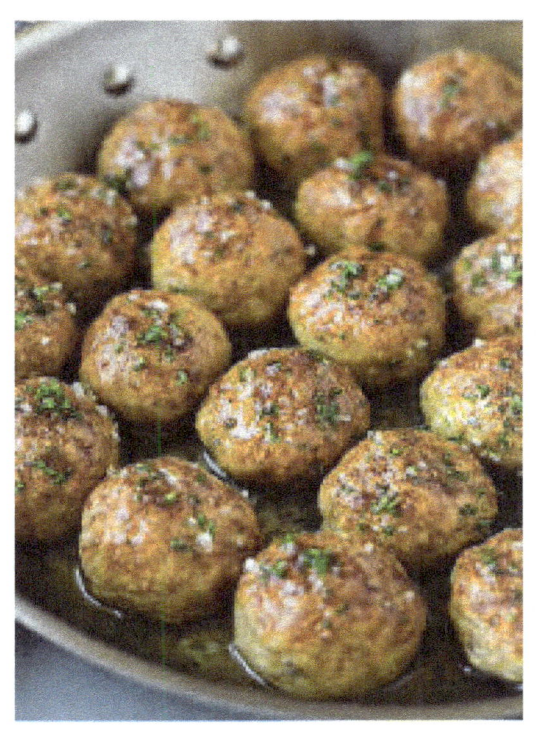

Easy Italian Meatballs

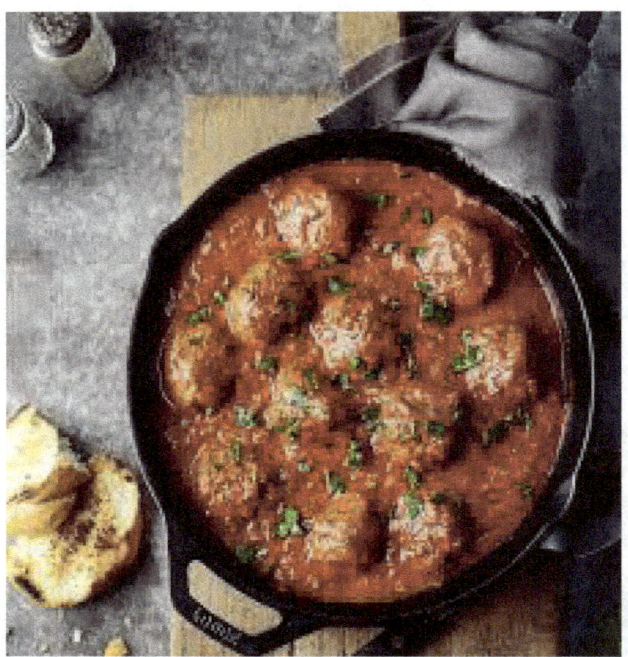

Basic Recipe
Preparation Time: 10 minutes
Cooking Time: 13 minutes
Serving: 4

Ingredients:

- 2-lb. lean ground turkey
- ¼ cup onion, minced
- 2 cloves garlic, minced
- 2 tablespoons parsley, chopped
- 2 eggs
- 1½ cup parmesan cheese, grated
- ½ teaspoon red pepper flakes
- ½ teaspoon Italian seasoning
- Salt and black pepper to taste

Directions:

1. Toss all the meatball ingredients in a bowl and mix well. Make small meatballs out this mixture and place them in the air fryer basket.
2. Press "Power Button" of Air Fry Oven and turn the dial to select the "Air Fry" mode. Press the Time button and again turn the dial to set the cooking time to 13 minutes. Now push the Temp button and rotate the dial to set the temperature at 350 degrees F.
3. Once preheated, place the air fryer basket inside and close its lid.
4. Flip the meatballs when cooked halfway through.
5. Serve warm.

Nutrition: Calories 472 Fat 25.8 Carbs 1.7 g Protein 59.6 g

Oregano Chicken Breast

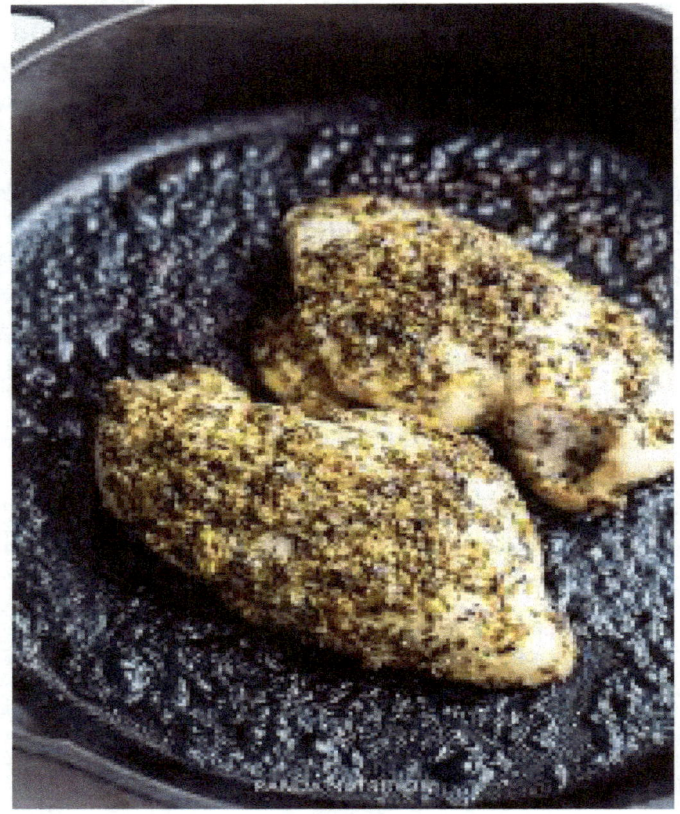

Basic Recipe
Preparation Time: 10 minutes
Cooking Time: 25 minutes
Serving: 6
Ingredients:
- 2 lbs. chicken breasts, minced
- 1 tablespoon avocado oil
- 1 teaspoon smoked paprika
- 1 teaspoon garlic powder
- 1 teaspoon oregano

- 1/2 teaspoon salt
- Black pepper, to taste

Directions:

1. Toss all the meatball ingredients in a bowl and mix well. Make small meatballs out this mixture and place them in the air fryer basket.
2. Press "Power Button" of Air Fry Oven and turn the dial to select the "Air Fry" mode. Press the Time button and again turn the dial to set the cooking time to 25 minutes
3. Now push the Temp button and rotate the dial to set the temperature at 375 degrees F.
4. Once preheated, place the air fryer basket inside and close its lid.
5. Serve warm.

Nutrition: Calories 352 Fat 14 g Carbs: 15.8 g Protein 26 g

Lemon Chicken Breasts

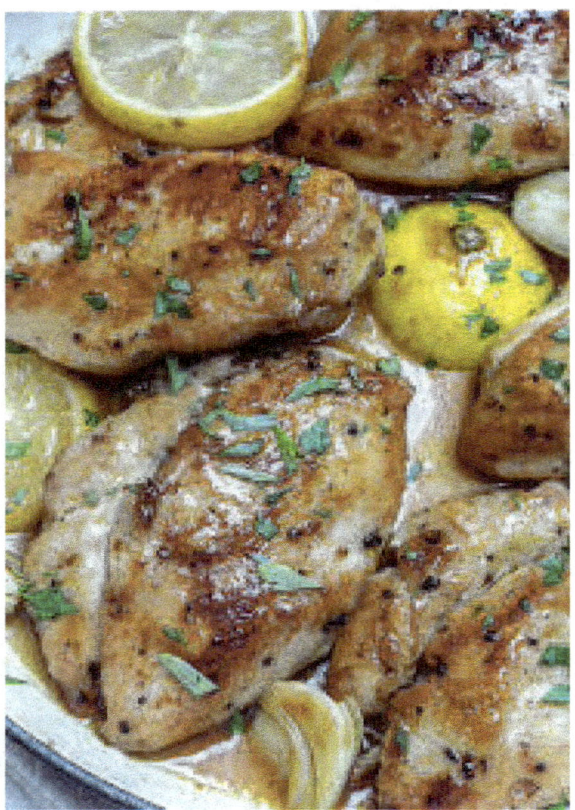

Basic Recipe
Preparation Time: 10 minutes
Cooking Time: 30 minutes
Serving: 4

Ingredients:

- 1/4 cup olive oil
- 3 tablespoons garlic, minced
- 1/3 cup dry white wine
- 1 tablespoon lemon zest, grated
- 2 tablespoons lemon juice
- 1 1/2 teaspoons dried oregano, crushed

- 1 teaspoon thyme leaves, minced
- Salt and black pepper
- 4 skin-on boneless chicken breasts
- 1 lemon, sliced

Directions:

1. Whisk everything in a baking pan to coat the chicken breasts well.
2. Place the lemon slices on top of the chicken breasts.
3. Spread the mustard mixture over the toasted bread slices.
4. Press "Power Button" of Air Fry Oven and turn the dial to select the "Bake" mode.
5. Press the Time button and again turn the dial to set the cooking time to 30 minutes
6. Now push the Temp button and rotate the dial to set the temperature at 370 degrees F.
7. Once preheated, place the baking pan inside and close its lid.
8. Serve warm.

Nutrition: Calories 388 Fat 8 g Carbs 8 g Protein 13 g

Cajun Salmon

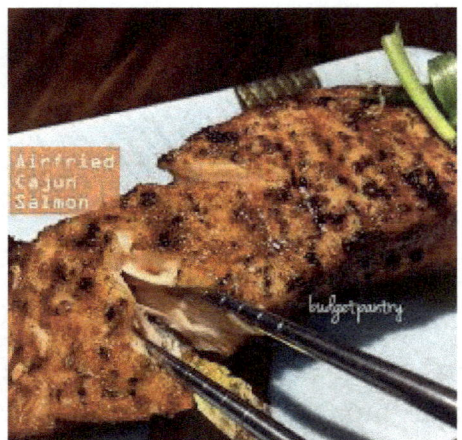

Basic Recipe
Preparation Time: 5 minutes
Cooking Time: 10 minutes
Serving: 2

Ingredients:

- 2 Salmon steaks
- 2 tbspcajun seasoning

Directions:

1. Rub the salmon steaks with the Cajun seasoning evenly. Set aside for about 10 minutes. Arrange the salmon steaks onto the greased cooking tray.
2. Arrange the drip pan in the bottom of the Instant Vortex Air Fryer Oven cooking chamber. Select "Air Fry" and then adjust the temperature to 390 °F. Set the time for 8 minutes and press "Start".
3. When the display shows "Add Food" insert the cooking tray in the center position. When the display shows "Turn Food" turn the salmon steaks.
4. When the cooking time is complete, remove the tray from the Vortex Oven. Serve hot.

Nutrition:
Calories 225 Carbs 0g Fat 10.5g Protein 22.1g

Buttered Salmon

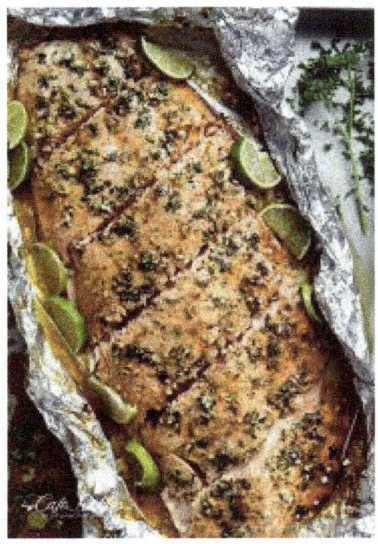

Basic Recipe
Preparation Time: 5 minutes
Cooking Time: 10 minutes
Serving: 2

Ingredients:
- 2 salmon fillets (6-oz)
- Salt and ground black pepper, as required
- 1 tbspbutter, melted

Directions:
1. Season each salmon fillet with salt and black pepper and then, coat with the butter. Arrange the salmon fillets onto the greased cooking tray.
2. Arrange the drip pan in the bottom of the Instant Vortex Air Fryer Oven cooking chamber. Select "Air Fry" and then adjust the temperature to 360 °F. Set the time for 10 minutes and press "Start".

3. When the display shows "Add Food" insert the cooking tray in the center position. When the display shows "Turn Food" turn the salmon fillets.
4. When cooking time is complete, remove the tray from the Vortex Oven. Serve hot.

Nutrition: Calories 276 Carbs 0g Fat 16.3g Protein 33.1g

CONCLUSION

Air fryers are a relatively new piece of kitchen gadgetry. They are used by individuals who want to cook healthy foods using less oil and less fat then their conventional counterparts.

In addition to being a healthier alternative to deep frying, air fryers are also fun to use. Air-frying not only produces lots of fun and tasty food, it also saves you time and money. You can cook without the need of a griddle or a stovetop, which frees up your kitchen so you can focus on eating more healthy foods!

It is important to have an air fryer that is up to par. If you want an air fryer that will last for years, make sure that you buy an durable one. To help you choose the right air fryer for you, we have compiled a list of the best air fried ovens!

The Airfryer has several seating options. The four different versions include:

Small Seating—The size of the seating area is 13.5" x 8.5" x 9.5".

Medium Seating—The size of the seating area is 20" x 12".

Large Seating—The size of the seating area is 23" x 15".

Extra Large Seating—The size is 32" X 21". The extra large seat could accommodate up to 8 pieces. A small, medium or large fryer is included with every air fryer and can be purchased separately. The only part that may need to be purchased separately is a colander for the basket which will hold up to 16 cups depending on the size of the basket that you are using. There are no other accessories required for the air fryer: please see the specifications on this page for further details.

What's happening to our restaurant food? The answer is rather simple. We are over-cooking and over-frying foods, and most of it is for the wrong reasons.

Nobody wants to eat overcooked, undercooked, or under-salted food. Restaurant owners are turning away good customers in the name of profit.

That's not our fault. It's up to the professional chefs to do a better job with their cooking skills.

We use our Air Fryers to cook foods that don't require cooking at all. We use them to cook and heat our foods in such a way that they're ready to eat right out of the air fryer. There's no need for you to heat up your kitchen with a conventional oven or stove, just put the food in and let it finish fully. You'll be amazed at how delicious your foods can taste when you use an Air Fryer!

Today's busy lifestyle often leaves us with little time to cook. For those of you who don't have time to cook, but still need your food, the air fryer is for you.

An air fryer is an appliance that cooks food by circulating hot air over it. The circulating air causes the food to slowly cook within a sealed container while removing excess oil and fat from the food. By sealing the food in a hermetic chamber during cooking, no additional oil is released into the air. This is important because it prevents the flavor of the food from being compromised. The result is a fast and easy way to prepare delicious meals without having to use any grease or oils while eroding your pantry of oils.

In this air fryer cookbook, we will teach you how to use your air fryer most effectively and how to avoid common mistakes. From learning how to clean and maintain your air fryer to finding creative recipes, this guide will help you get the most out of your air fryer today